Intensive Care Unit in Disaster

Editors

MARIE R. BALDISSERI
MARY JANE REED
RANDY S. WAX

CRITICAL CARE CLINICS

www.criticalcare.theclinics.com

Consulting Editor
JOHN A. KELLUM

October 2019 • Volume 35 • Number 4

ELSEVIER

1600 John F. Kennedy Boulevard • Suite 1800 • Philadelphia, Pennsylvania, 19103-2899

http://www.theclinics.com

CRITICAL CARE CLINICS Volume 35, Number 4
October 2019 ISSN 0749-0704, ISBN-13: 978-0-323-68391-3

Editor: Colleen Dietzler
Developmental Editor: Casey Potter

Critical Care Clinics (ISSN: 0749-0704) is published quarterly by Elsevier Inc., 360 Park Avenue South, New York, NY 10010-1710. Months of issue are January, April, July, and October. Business and Editorial Offices: 1600 John F. Kennedy Blvd., Suite 1800, Philadelphia, PA 19103-2899. Customer Service Office: 6277 Sea Harbor Drive, Orlando, FL 32887-4800. Periodicals postage paid at New York, NY and additional mailing offices. Subscription prices are $243.00 per year for US individuals, $650.00 per year for US institution, $100.00 per year for US students and residents, $285.00 per year for Canadian individuals, $815.00 per year for Canadian institutions, $315.00 per year for international individuals, $815.00 per year for international institutions and $150.00 per year for Canadian and foreign students/residents. To receive student/resident rate, orders must be accompanied by name of affiliated institution, date of term, and the signature of program/residency coordinator on institution letterhead. Orders will be billed at individual rate until proof of status is received. Foreign air speed delivery is included in all *Clinics* subscription prices. All prices are subject to change without notice. POSTMASTER: Send address changes to *Critical Care Clinics*, Elsevier Periodicals Customer Service, 11830 Westline Industrial Drive, St. Louis, MO 63146. **Customer Service: 1-800-654-2452 (US). From outside of the US, call 1-314-447-8871. Fax: 1-314-447-8029. E-mail: journalscustomerservice-usa@ elsevier.com (for print support) or journalsonlinesupport-usa@elsevier.com (for online support).**

Reprints. For copies of 100 or more of articles in this publication, please contact the Commercial Reprints Department, Elsevier Inc., 360 Park Avenue South, New York, NY 10010-1710. Tel.: 212-633-3874; Fax: 212-633-3820; E-mail: reprints@elsevier.com.

Critical Care Clinics is also published in Spanish by Editorial Inter-Medica, Junin 917, 1er A, 1113, Buenos Aires, Argentina.

Critical Care Clinics is covered in *MEDLINE/PubMed (Index Medicus), EMBASE/Excerpta Medica, Current Concepts/Clinical Medicine, ISI/BIOMED, and Chemical Abstracts.*

Contributors

CONSULTING EDITOR

JOHN A. KELLUM, MD, MCCM
Professor, Critical Care Medicine, Medicine, Bioengineering and Clinical and Translational Science, Director, Center for Critical Care Nephrology, Vice Chair for Research, Department of Critical Care Medicine, University of Pittsburgh School of Medicine, Pittsburgh, Pennsylvania, USA

EDITORS

MARIE R. BALDISSERI, MD, MPH, FCCM
Professor of Critical Care Medicine and Neurocritical Care Medicine, University of Pittsburgh Medical Center, Department of Critical Care Medicine, Pittsburgh, Pennsylvania, USA

MARY JANE REED, MD, FACS, FCCM, FCCP
Director of Biocontainment Unit, Director of Neuroscience ICU, Departments of Critical Care Medicine and General Surgery, Geisinger Medical Center, Danville, Pennsylvania, USA

RANDY S. WAX, MD, MEd, FRCPC, FCCM
Staff Intensivist, Department of Critical Care Medicine, Medical Director, Academic Affairs, Lakeridge Health, Associate Professor, Department of Critical Care Medicine, Regional Director, Clinical Education, Lakeridge/Durham Clinical Hub, Faculty of Health Sciences, Queen's University, Oshawa, Ontario, Canada

AUTHORS

NEILL K.J. ADHIKARI, MSc
Associate Professor, Institute for Health Policy, Management and Evaluation, Dalla Lana School of Public Health, University of Toronto, Interdepartmental Division of Critical Care Medicine, University of Toronto, Sunnybrook Research Institute, Sunnybrook Hospital, Toronto, Ontario, Canada

AMADO ALEJANDRO BAEZ, MD, MSc, MPH
Department of Emergency Medicine/Center for Operational Medicine, Medical College of Georgia, Augusta University, Augusta, Georgia, USA; Postgraduate Studies, Universidad Nacional Pedro Henriquez Urena, Santo Domingo, Dominican Republic

MICHAEL D. CHRISTIAN, MD, MSc, FRCPC
Research and Clinical Effectiveness Lead, London's Air Ambulance, Bart's Health NHS Trust, Helipad, Royal London Hospital, London, United Kingdom

TIMOTHY M. DEMPSEY, MD, MPH
Assistant Professor of Medicine, Division of Pulmonary and Critical Care Medicine, Mayo Clinic, Rochester, Minnesota, USA

MICHAEL A. DEVITA, MD, FCCM, FRCP, FACP
Professor, Internal Medicine, Columbia University Vagelos College of Physicians and Surgeons, Harlem Hospital, New York, New York, USA

JEFFREY R. DICHTER, MD
Pulmonary, Allergy, Critical Care and Sleep Medicine, Associate Professor, University of Minnesota, Minneapolis, Minnesota, USA

DAVID J. DRIES, MSE, MD
Chair, Department of Surgery, Regions Hospital, HealthPartners Medical Group, Professor of Surgery and Emergency Medicine, University of Minnesota, Minneapolis, Minnesota, USA

SHARON EINAV, MSc, MD
Professor of Anesthesiology and Critical Care, Hebrew University Faculty of Medicine and Director of Surgical Intensive Care, Shaare Zedek Medical Center, Jerusalem, Israel

ROBERT A. FOWLER, MS (Epi)
Professor, Institute for Health Policy, Management and Evaluation, Dalla Lana School of Public Health, University of Toronto, Interdepartmental Division of Critical Care Medicine, University of Toronto, Sunnybrook Research Institute, Sunnybrook Hospital, Toronto, Ontario, Canada

JAMES GEILING, MD, MPH
Dartmouth Geisel School of Medicine, Hanover, New Hampshire, USA; Medical Service, VA Medical Center, White River Junction, Vermont, USA

MARYA GHAZIPURA, PhD(c), MS
Department of Population Health, New York University Langone Medical Center, New York, New York, USA

RAMON E. GIST, MD
Department of Pediatrics, Division of Pediatric Critical Care Medicine, SUNY Downstate Medical Center, Brooklyn, New York, USA

MITCHELL HAMELE, MD, LTC
Department of Pediatrics-Critical Care, Tripler Army Medical Center, Honolulu, Hawaii, USA

JORGE HIDALGO, MD, MACP, MCCM
Head of the Division of Critical Care, Karl Heusner Memorial Hospital, Belize, Central America

TANZIB HOSSAIN, MD, MS
Pulmonary and Critical Care Fellow, New York University Langone Medical Center, New York, New York, USA

CHRISTINA M. JAMROS, DO
Division of Infectious Diseases, Department of Internal Medicine, Naval Medical Center, San Diego, California, USA

DAVID A. KAPPEL, MD, FACS
Clinical Professor of Surgery, West Virginia University School of Medicine, Deputy Medical Director, WVOEMS, West Virginia State Trauma System, Wheeling, West Virginia, USA

PETER KIIZA, MBChB, DTM&H
Research Fellow, Sunnybrook Research Institute, Sunnybrook Hospital, Toronto, Ontario, Canada

NIRANJAN KISSOON, MD
Department of Pediatrics and Emergency Medicine, BC Children's Hospital, Sunny Hill Health Centre for Children, UBC, Clinical Investigator, Child and Family Research Institute, Vancouver, British Columbia, Canada

STEPHANIE C. LAPINSKY, BSc, MD
Division of Critical Care Medicine, University of Toronto, Toronto, Ontario, Canada

STEPHEN E. LAPINSKY, MB BCh, MSc, FRCPC
Division of Critical Care Medicine, University of Toronto, Toronto, Ontario, Canada

RYAN C. MAVES, MD
Program Director, Infectious Diseases Fellowship, Faculty Physician, Critical Care Medicine Service, Department of Internal Medicine, Naval Medical Center, San Diego, California, USA

ERIC MELNYCHUK, DO
Department of Critical Care Medicine, Geisinger Medical Center, Danville, Pennsylvania, USA

BUSHRA MINA, MD, FCCM, FCCP, FACP
Director of Fellowship Program, Pulmonary and Critical Care Division, Lenox Hill Hospital, Northwell Health, New York, New York, USA

RASHMI MISHRA, MD
Pulmonary Critical Care Physician, The Lung Center, Penn Highlands Healthcare, DuBois, Pennsylvania, USA

MICHAEL JAMES ELLETT MONSON, LCDR
Department of Pulmonary and Critical Care Medicine, Naval Medical Center San Diego, San Diego, California, USA

SARAH MULLIN, BSc(candidate)
Student, Department of Psychology, Faculty of Health, York University, Toronto, Ontario, Canada

ALEXANDER S. NIVEN, MD
Associate Professor of Medicine, Mayo Clinic College of Medicine and Science, Division of Pulmonary and Critical Care Medicine, Mayo Clinic, Rochester, Minnesota, USA

MALY ORON, MD
Pulmonary and Critical Care Division, Lenox Hill Hospital, Northwell Health, New York, New York, USA

JOHN S. PARRISH, MD
Department of Pulmonary and Critical Care Medicine, Naval Medical Center San Diego, San Diego, California, USA

SHALIN PATEL, MD
MedStar Georgetown University Hospital/MedStar Montgomery Medical Center, Olney, Maryland, USA

MICHAEL POWERS, MD, LCDR, MC, USN
Department of Pulmonary and Critical Care Medicine, Director, Pulmonary Function Test Lab, Assistant Program Director, Pulmonary and Critical Care Medicine Fellowship, Assistant Professor of Medicine, Naval Medical Center San Diego, San Diego, California, USA

MARY JANE REED, MD, FACS, FCCM, FCCP
Director of Biocontainment Unit, Director of Neuroscience ICU, Departments of Critical Care Medicine and General Surgery, Geisinger Medical Center, Danville, Pennsylvania, USA

VALERIE BRIDGET SATKOSKE, MSW, PhD
Assistant Professor, West Virginia University School of Medicine, Wheeling Hospital, Wheeling, West Virginia, USA

GILBERT SEDA, MD, PhD
Department of Pulmonary and Critical Care Medicine, Naval Medical Center San Diego, San Diego, California, USA

ALFRED G. SMITH, DO
Division of Infectious Diseases, Department of Internal Medicine, Naval Medical Center, San Diego, California, USA

KOREN TEO, BScPHM, MHSc
Captain, Canadian Forces Health Services Group, Toronto, Ontario, Canada

MACIEJ WALCZYSZYN, MD
Director, Pulmonary and Critical Care Division, Flushing Hospital Medical Center, Flushing, New York, USA

RANDY S. WAX, MD, MEd, FRCPC, FCCM
Staff Intensivist, Department of Critical Care Medicine, Medical Director, Academic Affairs, Lakeridge Health, Associate Professor, Department of Critical Care Medicine, Regional Director, Clinical Education, Lakeridge/Durham Clinical Hub, Faculty of Health Sciences, Queen's University, Oshawa, Ontario, Canada

FREDERIC S. ZIMMERMAN, MD
Department of Intensive Care, Shaare Zedek Medical Center, Jerusalem, Israel

Contents

The "daily disasters" within the ebb and flow of routine critical care provide a foundation of preparedness for the less-frequent, larger events that affect most health care organizations at some time. Although large disasters can overwhelm, those who strengthen processes and habits through daily practice will be the best prepared to manage them.

Critical care teams can face a dramatic surge in demand for ICU beds and organ support during a disaster. Through effective preparedness, teams can enable a more effective response and hasten recovery back to normal operations. Disaster preparedness needs to balance an all-hazards approach with focused hazard-specific preparation guided by a critical care-specific hazard-vulnerability analysis. Broad stakeholder input from within and outside the critical care team is necessary to avoid gaps in planning. Evaluation of critical care disaster plans require frequent exercises, with a mechanism in place to ensure lessons learned effectively prompt improvements in the plan.

A health care facility must develop a comprehensive disaster plan that has a provision for critical care services. Mass critical care requires surge capacity: augmentation of critical care services during a disaster. Surge capacity involves staff, supplies, space, and structure. Measures to increase critical care staff include recalling essential personnel, using noncritical care staff, and emergency credentialing of volunteers. Having an adequate supply chain and a cache of critical care supplies is essential. Virtual critical care or tele-critical care can augment critical care capacity by assisting with patient monitoring, specialized consultation, and in pandemics reduces staff exposure.

This review provides an overview of triaging critically ill or injured patients during mass casualty incidents due to events such as disasters, pandemics, or terrorist incidents. Questions clinicians commonly have, including "what is triage?," "when to triage?," "what are the types of disaster

providers. Patients may make complete recovery with aggressive support- ive care, even if they appear to have a poor prognosis. Hospitals must have an emergency response disaster plan in place to deal with all potential causes of disasters, including illnesses resulting from chemical agents.

systems. Previous outbreaks offer lessons for health system preparedness and response, including establishment of hospital-based high-risk pathogen treatment units. Their creation demands early preparation and interprofessional coordination; infection prevention and control; case management training; prepositioning of supplies; conversion of existing structures to treatment units; and strengthening communication and research platforms. Hospital-based Ebola and high-risk pathogen treatment units may improve case detection, interrupt transmission, and improve staff safety and patient care.

In preparation for Superstorm Sandy, the emergency control center at Lenox Hill Hospital (LHH) was activated. Patients were evacuated safely to increase hospital capacity, including increased critical care beds, hospital equipment and supplies, including ventilators. A triage center was established in the emergency department at LHH. Efforts were coordinated between LHH and New York University (NYU) Langone Medical Center. NYU medical staff was granted Disaster Emergency privileges, credentialed at LHH, and oriented to LHH. NYU residents and fellows were added by the Office of Graduate Medical Education.

Emergency and critical care medicine are fraught with ethically challenging decision making for clinicians, patients, and families. Time and resource constraints, decisional-impaired patients, and emotionally overwhelmed family members make obtaining informed consent, discussing withholding or withdrawing of life-sustaining treatments, and respecting patient values and preferences difficult. When illness or trauma is secondary to disaster, ethical considerations increase and change based on number of casualties, type of disaster, and anticipated life cycle of the crisis. This article considers the ethical issues that arise when health providers are confronted with the challenges of caring for victims of disaster.

CRITICAL CARE CLINICS

SERIES OF RELATED INTEREST

Emergency Medicine Clinics
Available at: https://www.emed.theclinics.com/

THE CLINICS ARE AVAILABLE ONLINE!
Access your subscription at:
www.theclinics.com

Preface
Critical State of Disaster Preparedness

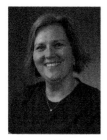
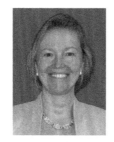
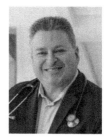

Marie R. Baldisseri, MD,
MPH, FCCM

Mary Jane Reed, MD, FACS,
FCCM, FCCP

Randy S. Wax, MD, MEd,
FRCPC, FCCM

Editors

Disasters both natural and anthropogenic are increasing in intensity and frequency. 2018 marked the eighth consecutive year in which greater than seven high-consequence natural disasters occurred in the United States alone. These numbers do not include mass shootings or disease outbreaks, such as measles, influenza, and hepatitis A.

Unfortunately, our health care systems, which are already overburdened, undersupported, and in some cases nonexistent, are often unprepared for a sudden surge of patients or substantial infrastructure failure. Disasters overwhelm local capacity, leading to sudden or gradual decline of the health of a community. Preparing for disaster is foremost in a community's priority at the time of the disaster and immediately after. For a variety of reasons, disaster preparedness awareness during normal operations can wane, leading to inadequate preparedness. The 2019 US National Health Security Preparedness Index, which assesses the ability to provide health care in large-scale public threats, revealed only a moderate level of overall preparedness with a score of 6.7 out of 10. However, the metric measuring the ability to maintain quality health care during the event and after was only 4.9, revealing a significant gap in preparedness.[1]

Intensive care units (ICUs) and providers should be on the frontlines of disaster planning as most of the injuries and pathologies of today's disasters often need higher level of care. Critical care providers also have experience in triage and utilization of resources. The editors of this publication have given a broad overview of considerations for ICU preparation as well as specific examples of how others have confronted significant threats to health security for their critically ill patients. Our hope in bringing these expert authors together is to motivate our colleagues and all stakeholders to make disaster preparedness a priority in their hospitals and practices.

Marie R. Baldisseri, MD, MPH, FCCM
Department of Critical Care Medicine
University of Pittsburgh Medical Center
3550 Terrace Street
Pittsburgh, PA 15213, USA

Mary Jane Reed, MD, FACS, FCCM, FCCP
Department of Critical Care Medicine
Geisinger Medical Center
100 North Academy Avenue
Danville, PA 17822-2037, USA

Randy S. Wax, MD, MEd, FRCPC, FCCM
Department of Critical Care Medicine
Lakeridge Health
Department of Critical Care Medicine
Queen's University
1 Hospital Court
Oshawa, ON L1G 2B9, Canada

E-mail addresses:
baldisserimr@ccm.upmc.edu (M.R. Baldisseri)
mreed@geisinger.edu (M.J. Reed)
randy.wax@queensu.ca (R.S. Wax)

REFERENCE

1. National Health Security Preparedness Index. Update National Health Security Index 2019. Robert Wood Johnson Foundation. Available at: https://nhspi.org/. Accessed July 5, 2019.

Intensive Care Role in Disaster Management Critical Care Clinics

Tanzib Hossain, MD, MS[a], Marya Ghazipura, PhD(c), MS[b],
Jeffrey R. Dichter, MD[c],*

KEYWORDS

- Disaster preparedness • Conventional, contingency, and crisis care • Surge capacity
- ICU strain • Prioritization • Triage

KEY POINTS

- Mass disasters require governmental, administrative, and clinical planning, and it is quite important for intensivist expertise be involved in disaster preparedness at all levels.
- Intensive care unit (ICU) surge capacity may be considered a spectrum from conventional daily care (up to 120% hospital capacity) through contingency and ultimately crisis care (>200% above hospital capacity).
- ICU strain is a test of ICU surge capacity, with (near) capacity ICU census and increasing admission wait time foremost among admission strain measures given their direct impact on rising mortality. Other strain measures include patient turnover, patients transferred out of hospital or declined ICU admission due to lack of ICU beds, acuity of illness, and nurse-to-patient ratio. Discharge strain indicators include "after-hours" transfers, which are associated with increased mortality and ICU readmissions.

Continued

DEFINING DISASTER

Caring for the critically ill or injured due to disasters has only increased in need as disasters have evolved over time and the vulnerability of societies to their effects has been maintained.[1–3] Defining what is meant by a "disaster" is paramount toward

Disclosures: T. Hossain, J.R. Dichter, and M. Ghazipura have no financial conflicts of interest to disclose regarding this article. T. Hossain and J.R. Dichter are members of the Task Force for Mass Critical Care, an academic group composed of critical care professionals who do research in disaster preparedness.
[a] New York University Langone Medical Center, 462 First Avenue, 7N24, New York, NY 10016, USA; [b] Department of Population Health, New York University Langone Medical Center, 330 East 39th Street, Suite 26B, New York, NY 10016, USA; [c] Pulmonary, Allergy, Critical Care and Sleep Medicine, University of Minnesota, MMC 276, 420 Delaware Street SE, Minneapolis, MN 55455, USA
* Corresponding author.
E-mail address: jdichter@umn.edu

Continued

- Response strategies for ICU strain under conventional daily care include prioritization of patients awaiting ICU admission, responsible ICU discharge of patients at the earliest opportunity, consideration for initiating a focused incident command center to help facilitate rapid admission of patients to the ICU, and hospital transfer of patients when timely ICU care cannot be provided.
- The response strategies for contingency and crisis care are based on the principles for conventional daily care, but greater in scope, and often use strategies including conserve, substitute, adapt, reuse, reallocate, and triage of scarce resources.

preparing for and managing the consequences. What constitutes a disaster has evolved over time from strict quantitative parameters to focusing on social disruption.[4] During this period, disasters have been defined in a variety of ways by various stakeholders involved with disaster response (**Table 1**).[5–8] Ultimately, it is necessary to take into account multiple different definitions in order to fully encapsulate the wide-ranging effects of disasters.

The common theme among definitions is that a disaster disrupts normal function and causes suffering and loss that exceed the capacity of a region to cope. In most

Table 1
Definitions of disasters

Source	Definition
International	
United Nations (UN SPIDER)	Disruption of function causing widespread losses exceeding the ability for a society to cope using its own resources
World Health Organization (WHO)	An occurrence disrupting the normal conditions of existence and causing a level of suffering that exceeds the capacity of adjustment of the affected community
International Federation of the Red Cross/Crescent (IFRC)	A sudden, calamitous event that seriously disrupts the functioning of a community or society and causes human, material, and economic or environmental losses that exceed the community's or society's ability to cope using its own resources
United States	
Federal Emergency Management Association (FEMA)	An occurrence that has resulted in property damage, deaths, or injuries to a community
US Stafford Act	Any natural catastrophe, or, regardless of cause, any fire, flood, or explosion, in any part of the United States, which in the determination of the president causes damage of sufficient severity and magnitude to warrant major disaster assistance under this act to supplement the efforts and available resources of states, local governments, and disaster relief organizations in alleviating the damage, loss, hardship, or suffering caused thereby

Data from Refs.[5–8]

instances, emergency personnel with additional resources are then redirected to these areas. In the United States, the Stafford Act states, emergency response providers include "Federal, State, and local governmental and nongovernmental emergency public safety, fire, law enforcement, emergency response, emergency medical (including hospital emergency facilities), and related personnel, agencies, and authorities."[6] The Act then states that these entities are responsible for identifying "evacuation modes and capabilities, including the use of mass and public transit capabilities, and coordinating and integrating evacuation plans for all populations, including for those individuals located in hospitals, nursing homes, and other institutional living facilities."[6]

Although the importance of planning for hospital evacuations is noted in the Act, what is missing in the preceding language is the additional role of hospital personnel and facilities outside of the emergency department (ED), in particular the intensive care units (ICU), in disaster response and management. The involvement of critical care personnel in both hospital and regional disaster preparedness and response committees and organizations is of vital importance for appropriate delivery of care for the critically ill in disasters.

For the critical care physician in charge of caring for critically ill patients throughout the hospital (both in and out of the ICU), the disaster-affected area becomes the entire hospital. Although preservation of hospital infrastructure entails (potential) allocation of scarce hospital resources, the overriding priority is to maintain patient care at a high level regardless of barriers presented by a disaster.

WHY CRITICAL CARE MEDICINE IS IMPORTANT IN DISASTER PREPAREDNESS

Although inside the walls of the ICU may be where most critical care is delivered, many important critical care services are provided urgently after an event or onset of illness outside of an ICU and hospital.[9] The role of intensivists is important in leading preparedness planning for events of this nature, and equally so in the clinical and organizational roles during a disaster event.[9]

Critical care leaders must provide leadership preparedness at the level of state departments of health, health system and hospital planning, and involvement in incident command centers during actual events. Planning includes system-level and site-level communication and sharing of resources, especially when nearing the point of limiting scarce resources; sharing of clinical expertise across organizations; and transportation of patients; among others.[1,9–14] Preparedness also requires planning for surge capacity of staff, ICU space, and supplies and medications across the spectrum of disaster severity from conventional to contingency and crisis (**Fig. 1**).[11,13,15]

Clinically, intensivists involved in resuscitation and ongoing care in transport have been recognized as crucial in preventing needless morbidity and death.[9] Critical care interfaces with other departments, especially the ED, are as important to ensure critical illness is recognized, treated, and admission to ICU expedited. Preparedness in addition means developing the ability to expand critical care capacity beyond the ICU in nonroutine ICU care areas, educating noncritical care staff how to assist in providing care ("force multipliers"), and planning for additional supplies and medication requirements.[9,10,12,14,15]

Finally, unlike other departments in the hospital, the demands on the ICU tend to be prolonged given it is the end-destination for critically ill patients with hospital stays lasting days to weeks longer than the event itself, rather than hours, as is the case in the ED. Therefore, surge planning needs to be able to account for a prolonged duration of ICU functioning at a given surge capacity.[11,14,16,17]

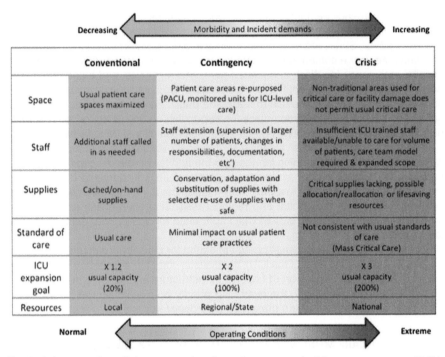

Fig. 1. A framework outlining conventional, contingency, and crisis surge responses. PACU, post-anesthesia care unit. (*From* Christian MD, Devereaux AV, Dichter JR. Introduction and executive summary: care of the critically ill and injured during pandemics and disasters: CHEST consensus statement. Chest. 2014 Oct;146(4 Suppl):8S–34S. https://doi.org/10.1378/chest.14-0732.)

HOW CRITICAL CARE EXPERTISE IS INTEGRAL IN DISASTER PREPAREDNESS AND RESPONSE
Conventional Care Conditions (up to 120% of Hospital Capacity)

ICUs by their nature face daily challenges, and the monthly/yearly "average volume" of patients does not account for the routine episodic surges of critical illness that place demands on a unit. These surges intensify the strain ICUs commonly face when running at or beyond capacity, given the dynamic of discharges and admissions when the resource needs exceed availability. These routine surges are indeed a test of *conventional* disaster preparedness, and routinely operate toward the boundary of contingency care, or up to 120% above hospital capacity[11,18] (see **Fig. 1**).

This article in *Critical Care Clinics* initially addresses surge capacity, also described as ICU strain, at the level of conventional care with focus on the impact on patient flow and development of strategies to optimize it. Although surge capacity is composed of space, staff, and supplies (including medications), under conventional circumstances the most important critical care resource are ICU beds whose components include both space limitations and the necessary professional staff (especially nursing) to support the beds.[11,18,19] The principles discussed herein are focused on an individual ICU, but can easily be integrated at a system level across ICUs, hospitals, and health systems.[10] Conventional care conditions, discussed first, also form the basis for contingency and crisis care.[18]

ICU strain may be defined as a dynamic discordance between available resources and demand to admit more critically ill patients while continuing to provide the highest quality, optimal care.[20–22] Strain can result in denied ICU admissions, and delayed admission from the ED and other areas with a corresponding increased risk of disability and death.[19,23–25] Strain also affects the decisions and actions of critical care professionals and may lead to premature ICU discharges, unplanned readmissions, and increased adverse events and mortality.[20–22]

ICU strain is described based on adapted admission and discharge strain indicators,[22] which also overlap with ICU quality measures[22,26–28] (**Table 2**). Among admission indicators, higher census is included given the association with higher acuity admissions and mortality,[21,29] with increased mortality up to 11.6% noted during periods of strain.[21] ICU admission wait time is included, particularly from the ED, as it too is associated with increased mortality (see discussion that follows).[23–25,30] Declined ICU admission, patient turnover, nurse-to-patient ratio, and transfers out of hospital due to lack of an ICU bed are included as common measures of ICU workload and capacity limit.[22] Discharge indicators include after-hours discharges and readmissions, all of which reflect the strain of releasing ICU patients early to increase capacity, and are associated with increased mortality (discussed later in this article).[19,22,31,32]

Table 2 ICU strain indicators with definitions and threshold levels of concern		
Strain Indicator	**Definition**	**Threshold Level of Concern**
Admission indicators		
Intensive care unit (ICU) census	% of bed ICU occupancy	85%–90%
Admission wait time (Queuing)	Time from ICU admission orders written until ICU patient arrival	≥4–6 h delay to ICU admission*
Patient turnover	The number of admissions and discharges in a 24-h period	No set standard, but higher consistent with greater strain
ICU transfers out of hospital due to lack of ICU beds	Inter-hospital transfers due to lack of an open ICU bed	>0
Declined admission to ICU	Number of patients (%) declined ICU admission compared with total number of consults due to lack of an ICU bed	>0
ICU acuity	Severity of illness measure (eg, SOFA, APACHE II scores)	Variable
Nurse-to-patient ratio	The number of patients per ICU nurse	1:1 to ≤2:1
Release indicators		
"After-hour" ICU releases	Unplanned release from ICU outside of regular hours (ICU-specific definition)	>0
ICU readmissions	Avoidable ICU readmission within 48 h of ICU discharge	>0

Abbreviations: APACHE, acute physiologic assessment and chronic health evaluation; ICU, intensive care unit; SOFA, sequential organ failure assessment.
Data from Refs.[22,26–28]

We recommend routine daily monitoring of admission and discharge strain indicators as a group, as each indicator reflects different yet important processes. More frequent monitoring of strain indicators is recommended during peak periods or during an ongoing disaster surge.

Strain indicators are intended to evoke 3 adaptive strategies in response to their urgency. In addition to these strategies, however, optimizing ICU quality patient care processes contributes not only to highest quality care, but also supports the most efficient operations during ICU stay, so their importance cannot be overstated. Although it is not the purpose of this article to review routine ICU care, some of the most important care processes include the ABCDEF bundle,[33–35] sepsis bundle,[36] teamwork, and daily multidisciplinary rounds,[37] among others.[28] These processes may provide potential benefits of decreased mortality, ICU and hospital length of stay, and decreased risk of ICU readmission.

Admission Strain Indicator Response Strategies

The first adaptive response strategy is prioritization of patients for ICU admission based on their level of acute needs and risk. The second strategy is admitting patients from the ED and other areas within a 4-hour to 6-hour window and ensuring they receive ongoing high-quality care in the transition process. Last is ensuring patients are transferred to other hospitals when it is evident they cannot receive the necessary care in a timely manner in the original strained facility. These 3 strategies are depicted in **Fig. 2**.

Prioritization for Admission

There are no established systematic criteria by which critically ill patients are *prioritized* for admission to an ICU. In approaching these decisions, Intensivists traditionally use criteria that include bed availability, severity of illness, code status, functional baseline, presence of comorbid conditions, and age, among others factors.[38] In addition, admission decisions are usually made with input from nursing and other disciplines.[39]

Using the Society of Critical Care Medicine (SCCM) admission, discharge, and triage guidelines as a basis, we recommend dividing patients seeking

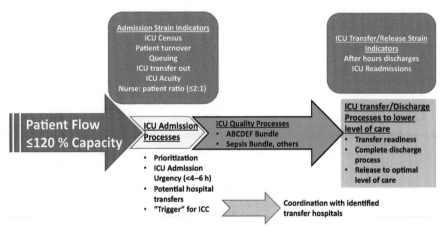

Fig. 2. ICU patient flow, conventional care: admission and discharge strain indicators with corresponding ICU admission processes, ICU quality processes, and ICU transfer/discharge processes. ICC, incident command center.

ICU admission into 2 priority levels (**Table 3**). Higher priority includes patients needing active life support for organ failure, including mechanical ventilation, vasopressors, invasive hemodynamic monitoring, and other such therapies. Higher-priority criteria also include specific clinical signs or metabolic derangements (column B) based in part on rapid response criteria and common experience, and may indeed represent higher-urgency patients who have not yet developed organ failure.[19,40]

Lower-priority patients are similar but have factors that may decrease the necessity or benefit of ICU care and may include limitations of care, such as directives placing restrictions on escalation of care, severe underlying illnesses, and/or poor functional baseline.[19] The use of severity scores has been placed in the lower-priority section, as most systems are validated as retrospective assessments rather than preadmission tools, and tend to predict ICU outcomes rather than relative benefit of ICU care.[19,41] Patients requiring observation only also would be considered lower priority. **Fig. 3** illustrates patients in both higher and lower-priority "buckets" placed on a priority "ladder" using these factors.

Our recommendation is to rely on intensivist clinical judgment with input from nursing and other appropriate professionals, to separate potential patients into higher

Table 3
Prioritization criteria for patients considered for ICU admission (see also Fig. 3)

Higher Priority	
A. Based on specific clinical needs	B. Based on specific clinical signs (VS) or laboratory data

Invasive support
• Mechanical ventilation
• Hemodynamic support and monitoring
• Continuous renal replacement therapy
• Therapies requiring aggressive monitoring and adjustments
• Significant metabolic derangements
	• Respiratory/Cardiovascular
	  ○ ↑ RR >26, ↑ HR >120
	  ○ ↓ SBP <100
	  ○ Increased work of breathing
	  ○ Potentially threatened airway
	  ○ Cyanosis or mottling
	• Neurologic deterioration
	  ○ Seizures, new focal deficit, delirium
	• Metabolic: ↑ Lactate or creatinine

Lower Priority	
• Limitations of care that significantly decrease potential benefit of ICU (no intubation; no cardiac resuscitation) • Presence of advanced malignancy, or severe chronic organ dysfunction • Functional baseline impairment before hospitalization • Patients requiring noninvasive support (eg, BIPAP) • Patients requiring observation only • Patients less likely to benefit from ICU care either because of very poor prognosis, or highly favorable prognosis irrespective of it	• Acuity score if available (SOFA, APACHE II, others)

Abbreviations: ↑, means elevated respiratory rate (RR); elevated heart rate (HR); ↓, means decreased systolic blood pressure (SBP); APACHE, acute physiologic assessment and chronic health evaluation; BIPAP, bilevel positive airway pressure; HR, heart rate; ICU, intensive care unit; RR, respiratory rate; SBP, systolic blood pressure; SOFA, sequential organ failure assessment; VS, vital signs.
Data from Refs.[19,39–41]

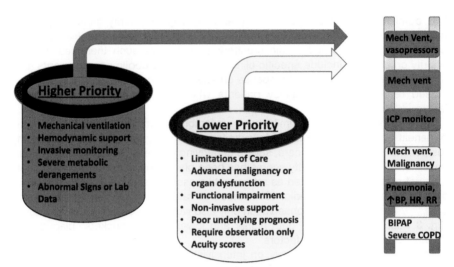

Fig. 3. Prioritization criteria for patients considered for ICU admission. Conventional and contingency care: illustration of higher-priority and lower-priority patient "buckets" and how example patients may be placed on the prioritization "ladder." BIPAP, bilevel positive airway pressure; BP, blood pressure; COPD, chronic obstructive pulmonary disease; HR, heart rate; ICP, intracranial pressure; Mech Vent, mechanical ventilation; RR, respiratory rate (*Data from* Refs.[19,39–41])

or lower-priority levels, and then further prioritizing within each level (see **Table 3**). Although most higher-priority patients may receive preference, there will undoubtedly be instances in which lower-priority patients may have greater urgency.

ICUs should have their own written processes to account for ICU admission prioritization.[19,41,42] These processes should be straightforward to implement under the duress of daily practice,[19,39,41] with the underlying guiding principle being highest prioritization for patients most likely to benefit from ICU care and whose chances for survival or a more functional outcome would be most compromised without it.[19,41]

Critically Ill Patients Waiting for Intensive Care Unit Admission

Critically ill patients waiting in the ED for ICU admission have increasing risk of mortality the longer they reside there.[23,24] Evidence further suggests this risk is present for surgical patients in post-anesthesia care areas, and patients in other hospital areas also awaiting ICU admission.[25,30] This risk is substantial, with an odds ratio (OR) of persistent organ dysfunction or death of 1.77 per hour ED boarding time, an OR 5.32 for post-anesthesia care unit patients waiting 6 hours or more, and a 1.5% increased risk of death per hour wait time for ward patients.[24,25,30] Although it is difficult to define precisely the degree of risk and duration of time at which point this risk rises, 4 to 6 hours is the recommended maximum time patients should wait outside the ICU before admission.[19,24] The etiology for this increasing risk is unknown, but its importance as a public health hazard has been identified.[43]

SCCM suggests that all hospitals have designated beds, staff, and supplies to support the critically ill in the event of a mass casualty incident,[19] and the Task Force for Mass Critical Care suggests that hospitals be able to surge immediately to at least 20% above hospital ICU capacity for a conventional event.[11] Given the rising mortality risk for patients waiting for ICU admission, it is therefore reasonable to use ICU queuing time as a "trigger" for a conventional-level disaster response (**Box 1**).

Box 1
Recommended trigger and conventional disaster response processes when patients in intensive care unit (ICU) admission queue exceed designated threshold

Trigger:
• Any patient waiting for an ICU bed >6 hours, or 2 patients waiting for more than 4 hours each.

Response:
• Initiating a focused incident command center (ICC) until patients awaiting ICU are dispositioned.
• Increasing critical care professional staffing for patients with pending ICU admission.
  ○ Nurse staffing ratio of 2:1 to ensure ICU level of care.
  ○ Ongoing intensivist consultation and care.
• Consider cancelling/postponing elective surgical cases if potential positive impact on ICU bed availability.
• Transfer process initiated to other facilities for patients not admitted in a timely manner.
• Implementation of other mass casualty surge processes should be considered at this time.

The triggered response should include implementation of an incident command center, limited in scope but focused on the objective of admitting patients quickly to an ICU. If ICU beds are not imminently available, transfer plans to other hospitals should be made, and consideration given for cancellation of elective surgeries or procedures to decrease strain on available beds.[10,19,44] The triggered response should be chosen based on each hospital/health system's circumstances, and we suggest it be strongly considered when at least 1 to 2 patients approach significant queuing time risk (>4–6 hours).

Transferring Patients to Other Hospitals

Although data are limited regarding adult transport outcomes, transporting critically ill patients is generally safe,[45,46] particularly when transported by critical care–trained, experienced paramedic crews.[47] Published data suggest an adverse event rate of 6.5% of transfers, with hypotension and hemodynamic instability and hypoxemia being most events. Patients most at risk are those demonstrating hemodynamic instability (relative risk 3.7) or those on mechanical ventilation (relative risk 1.7) before transfer, with longer duration of transport also demonstrating increased risk.[46] Less is known of pediatric ICU transfers, but published data support higher mortality when patients are transferred from a ward bed compared with the ED (OR 1.76), suggesting possible delay due to underrecognized clinical deterioration.[48]

When a decision is made to transfer a patient, the priority is transferring the patient as quickly as possible, preferably direct from the ED, and with shorter planned durations of transport when able.[46,48] Appropriate pretransfer planning should focus on potential fluid and vasopressor management en route for patients who have demonstrated hypotension or are on mechanical ventilation.[46]

Patient transfers normally happen along informal patterns with higher-resourced hospitals receiving more transfers, and we recommend establishing formal processes and relationships with usual transfer/referring hospitals. In an emergency, these patterns may be disrupted, as regional resources are increasingly strained.[10] Large numbers of patients can be safely transferred, but require careful planning, including standard evacuation tools, sufficient resources, and logistical support.[49,50] In one example, a 24-bed ICU relocated all patients safely and without complication in 1 day.[51]

Intensive Care Unit Discharge/Transfer Processes

There is often pressure to open beds during a strain period, frequently resulting in ICU patients being transferred earlier than planned, often after hours at night. Data demonstrate that after-hours ICU transfers are associated with increased risk of in-hospital mortality (OR 1.30–1.39) and ICU readmission (OR 1.30),[19,31,32] although weekend discharges have not demonstrated greater risk than weekdays.[19,32] The explanation for this is not entirely clear and likely institution specific.

Our recommendation for after-hours ICU transfers/discharges is to use a defined standard ICU transfer process for all patients irrespective of time of transfer (**Box 2**). This should include an intensivist release assessment, with input and support from other professionals, and prioritization of ICU transfers/discharges based on risk; transfer to intermediate care or telemetry (rather than a ward bed) for higher-risk patients; and adherence to a formal transfer/discharge process in which the accepting physician receives both a verbal report from the intensivist/transferring physician and completes a clinical assessment and transfer orders.

Contingency to Crisis Care Events (120% to ≥200% Above Hospital Capacity)

When an event pushes a hospital, health system, or region toward contingency and crisis, the principles, priorities, and processes outlined previously for conventional care remain largely the same, although the magnitude and response increase dramatically. The spectrum of surge capacity is depicted in **Fig. 4**, illustrating the escalating imbalance of decreasing available resources versus increasing demand for them as an event moves closer to crisis.[1]

As patient volume increases and demand for ICU care exceeds capacity, this triggers the need for a regional incident command system.[10] (**Fig. 5**) With large

---

Box 2
Recommended ICU transfer/discharge process to ensure timely, optimal, and safe ICU transfer to intermediate or ward beds

ICU transfer/discharge criteria (particularly for "after-hours" discharge)

- Early ICU transfers/discharges have a spectrum of clinical issues and those patients at lower risk should be transferred first.
  - Consider *scheduled* ICU transfer/discharge periods 2 or more times per day (morning, afternoon).

- Higher-risk patients transferred/discharged to a higher level of care (intermediate care or telemetry) rather than routine ward bed. Risk factors for readmission include the following:
  - Advancing age.
  - Present and number of comorbidities.
  - Ongoing requirements for organ support, or otherwise medically challenging patients.
  - High ICU admission severity of illness scores (when available).

- Have a formal written ICU transfer/discharge process followed for *every* patient, irrespective of time of discharge.
  - Include a verbal report from releasing to accepting physician.
  - A formal clinical assessment and transfer orders completed by accepting physician.
  - Consider an additional scheduled provider follow-up visit soon after ICU release (eg, within 4–6 hours).

- Patients are released to areas that have appropriate nursing staff to support level of need.

Data from Refs.[19,31,32]

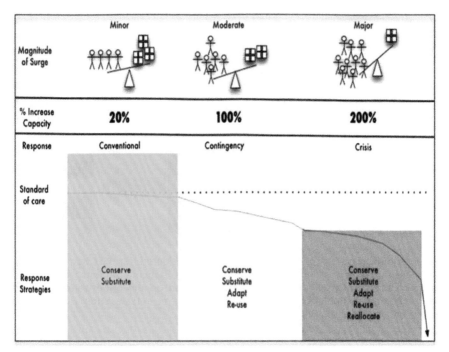

Fig. 4. Surge capacity across the spectrum of conventional, contingency, and crisis care. (*From* Christian MD, Devereaux AV, Dichter JR, et al. Introduction and executive summary: care of the critically ill and injured during pandemics and disasters: CHEST consensus statement. Chest. 2014 Oct;146(4 Suppl):8S–34S. https://doi.org/10.1378/chest.14-0732.)

events, local or state health departments may work with regional health care coalition partners to both communicate casualties and events, and coordinate care and transfers.[10] Slower-moving events (such as an evolving epidemic) may provide a chance for planning, whereas a sudden mass casualty incident may afford no

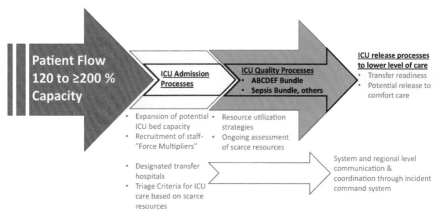

Fig. 5. ICU patient flow contingency and crisis care (120% to ≥ 200% capacity) and impact in altering changes on ICU admission processes, ICU care processes, and ICU transfer/discharge processes (changes in red).

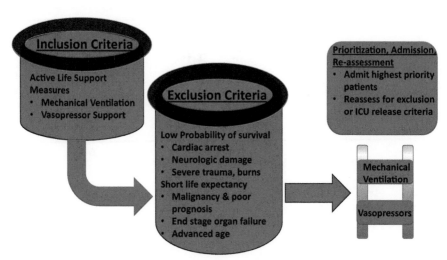

Fig. 6. Prioritization/triage criteria for patients considered for ICU admission: crisis care. Illustration of inclusion and exclusion priority patient "buckets" during crisis care, and the influence of which patients are placed on the prioritization "ladder," with ongoing scheduled reassessment for exclusion or release criteria. (*Data from* Refs.[1,19,39–41])

prior warning. Many of these types of events are discussed elsewhere in this publication.

The ICU resources of a hospital, health system, or region must be prepared to increase the capacity for ICU care, evaluate readiness for ICU and hospital discharges, and prioritize patients for admission[10,52] (see **Fig. 5**). Staffing for ICU care delivery in non-ICU areas including the ED and post-anesthesia care unit would be undertaken similarly to conventional care but in greater scale.[10,15,18] Resource conservation strategies including "conserve, substitute, adapt, reuse, and reallocate" would be initiated.[52] Patients would be transferred to other hospitals based on available capacity, with intent to optimally level the use of all available resources across the region.[10,15]

In a crisis-level event, prioritization may be even more urgent and intense, leading to scarce resource triage processes whereby those who may benefit most receiving the critical care resource whereas others are denied, with daily reassessment of priority.[1] The triage process includes narrowing inclusion criteria to mechanical ventilation and need for vasopressors and/or inotropes and establishing exclusion criteria based on low probability of survival and short life expectancy.[1] This focus on providing ICU-level care only to those with the greatest priority is depicted in **Fig. 6**.

SUMMARY

The "daily disasters" within the ebb and flow of routine critical care are the foundation of preparedness for the less frequent, larger events that affect most health care organizations at some time. Although these large events can overwhelm, the most prepared will be those who strengthen processes and habits through daily practice. The case study that follows is a particularly poignant example of the value of this preparedness.

Case Study: Prioritization and Triage, Bellevue Hospital During Hurricane Sandy, 2012

On October 29, 2012, Superstorm Sandy hit New York City, resulting in billions of dollars in damage and the shutdown of the nation's oldest public hospital, Bellevue.[53] Founded in 1736, Bellevue is an 828-bed level I trauma center with 56 adult ICU beds, and had survived other natural disasters, terrorist attacks, blackouts, the height of the AIDS epidemic, and the resurgence of tuberculosis in New York without having to evacuate patients and close its doors. Within 12 hours, this "behemoth" of a hospital was transformed into a building that could not sustain the care of its patients beyond a few days.

The hurricane flooding resulted in loss of water, communications, elevator services, suction, and oxygen. Soon after the storm started, the fuel pumps, located in the hospital basement and supplying the backup generators, flooded and failed, leaving sufficient fuel for only a few hours of operation. ICU preparations for this possibility included simplifying intravenous infusions and calculating infusion rates into drips per minute, having oxygen cylinders at bedsides, and having staff available to manually bag patients on ventilators.

There was concern at this point that only 1 smaller generator would remain functioning, supplying enough power for only 6 outlets in the ICU, and patients had to be evaluated and prioritized for who would receive the now critically scarce resource, electricity. Experience from Hurricane Irene in 2011 had led leadership to consider this very predicament, although power had not been lost in that situation. From that experience, however, strong clinical leadership led to the development of an ethical and transparent process for making the electricity allocation determinations using published guidelines. A multidisciplinary committee met that evening and reviewed each ICU patient based on severity of illness, need for life-sustaining therapy, and likelihood of recovery.

Power was ultimately sustained through heroic efforts from hospital staff and national guard troops who transported fuel drums up the stairways to the generators to keep them running. Although the need for drastic triage decisions were fortunately not necessary, the efforts of Bellevue leadership having the wisdom, drive, and courage in being prepared highlights and reinforces the importance of disaster planning.

REFERENCES

1. Christian MD, Sprung CL, King MA, et al. Triage: care of the critically ill and injured during pandemics and disasters: CHEST consensus statement. Chest 2014;146(4 Suppl):e61S–74S.

2. Degg M. Recent trends and future prospects. Geography 1992;77(336):198–209.

3. Rodriguez H, Donner W, Trainor J. Front matter. In: Rodriguez H, Donner W, Trainor J, editors. Handbook of disaster research. 2nd edition. Cham (Switzerland): Springer; 2018. p. i–xxxviii.

4. Perry R. Handbook of disaster research. In: Rodriguez H, Donner W, Trainor J, editors. Defining disaster: an evolving concept. 2nd edition. Cham (Switzerland): Springer; 2018. p. 3–22.

5. Portal UN-SK. Risks and disasters. 2019. Available at: http://www.un-spider.org/risks-and-disasters. Accessed April 30, 2019.

6. United States Code TTPHaW. Chapter 68. Disaster relief. Robert T. Stafford disaster relief and emergency assistance act 2018. Available at: https://www.

fema.gov/media-library-data/1519395888776-af5f95a1a9237302af7e3fd5b0d07
d71/StaffordAct.pdf. Accessed April 30, 2019.

7. Action WHOEH. Disasters and emergencies, definitions. Training package 2002. Available at: http://apps.who.int/disasters/repo/7656.pdf. Accessed April 30, 2019.

8. Cross IFotR. What is a disaster 2019. Available at: https://www.ifrc.org/en/what-we-do/disaster-management/about-disasters/what-is-a-disaster/. Accessed April 30, 2019.

9. Farmer JC, Carlton PK Jr. Providing critical care during a disaster: the interface between disaster response agencies and hospitals. Crit Care Med 2006;34(3 Suppl):S56–9.

10. Dichter JR, Kanter RK, Dries D, et al. System-level planning, coordination, and communication: care of the critically ill and injured during pandemics and disasters: CHEST consensus statement. Chest 2014;146(4 Suppl):e87S–102S.

11. Hick JL, Einav S, Hanfling D, et al. Surge capacity principles: care of the critically ill and injured during pandemics and disasters: CHEST consensus statement. Chest 2014;146(4 Suppl):e1S–16S.

12. Devereaux AV, Tosh PK, Hick JL, et al. Engagement and education: care of the critically ill and injured during pandemics and disasters: CHEST consensus statement. Chest 2014;146(4 Suppl):e118S–33S.

13. Parker MM. Critical care and disaster management. Crit Care Med 2006;34(3 Suppl):S52–5.

14. Shirley PJ, Mandersloot G. Clinical review: the role of the intensive care physician in mass casualty incidents: planning, organisation, and leadership. Crit Care 2008;12(3):214.

15. Einav S, Hick JL, Hanfling D, et al. Surge capacity logistics: care of the critically ill and injured during pandemics and disasters: CHEST consensus statement. Chest 2014;146(4 Suppl):e17S–43S.

16. Orban JC, Quintard H, Ichai C. ICU specialists facing terrorist attack: the Nice experience. Intensive Care Med 2017;43(5):683–5.

17. Gaarder C, Jorgensen J, Kolstadbraaten KM, et al. The twin terrorist attacks in Norway on July 22, 2011: the trauma center response. J Trauma Acute Care Surg 2012;73(1):269–75.

18. Hick JL, Barbera JA, Kelen GD. Refining surge capacity: conventional, contingency, and crisis capacity. Disaster Med Public Health Prep 2009;3(2 Suppl): S59–67.

19. Nates JL, Nunnally M, Kleinpell R, et al. ICU admission, discharge, and triage guidelines: a framework to enhance clinical operations, development of institutional policies, and further research. Crit Care Med 2016;44(8):1553–602.

20. Kerlin MP, Harhay MO, Vranas KC, et al. Objective factors associated with physicians' and nurses' perceptions of intensive care unit capacity strain. Ann Am Thorac Soc 2014;11(2):167–72.

21. Bagshaw SM, Wang X, Zygun DA, et al. Association between strained capacity and mortality among patients admitted to intensive care: a path-analysis modeling strategy. J Crit Care 2018;43:81–7.

22. Rewa OG, Stelfox HT, Ingolfsson A, et al. Indicators of intensive care unit capacity strain: a systematic review. Crit Care 2018;22(1):86.

23. Chalfin DB, Trzeciak S, Likourezos A, et al. Impact of delayed transfer of critically ill patients from the emergency department to the intensive care unit. Crit Care Med 2007;35(6):1477–83.

24. Mathews KS, Durst MS, Vargas-Torres C, et al. Effect of emergency department and ICU occupancy on admission decisions and outcomes for critically ill patients. Crit Care Med 2018;46(5):720–7.
25. Bing-Hua YU. Delayed admission to intensive care unit for critically surgical patients is associated with increased mortality. Am J Surg 2014;208(2):268–74.
26. Nouira H, Ben Abdelaziz A, Kacem M, et al. Which indicators are used to assess quality performance in intensive care units? A systematic review of medical literature. Anaesth Crit Care Pain Med 2018;37:583–7.
27. de Vos M, Graafmans W, Keesman E, et al. Quality measurement at intensive care units: which indicators should we use? J Crit Care 2007;22(4):267–74.
28. Murphy DJ, Ogbu OC, Coopersmith CM. ICU director data: using data to assess value, inform local change, and relate to the external world. Chest 2015;147(4):1168–78.
29. Gabler NB, Ratcliffe SJ, Wagner J, et al. Mortality among patients admitted to strained intensive care units. Am J Respir Crit Care Med 2013;188(7):800–6.
30. Cardoso LT, Grion CM, Matsuo T, et al. Impact of delayed admission to intensive care units on mortality of critically ill patients: a cohort study. Crit Care 2011;15(1):R28.
31. Vollam S, Dutton S, Lamb S, et al. Out-of-hours discharge from intensive care, in-hospital mortality and intensive care readmission rates: a systematic review and meta-analysis. Intensive Care Med 2018;44(7):1115–29.
32. Yang S, Wang Z, Liu Z, et al. Association between time of discharge from ICU and hospital mortality: a systematic review and meta-analysis. Crit Care 2016;20(1):390.
33. Balas MC, Vasilevskis EE, Olsen KM, et al. Effectiveness and safety of the awakening and breathing coordination, delirium monitoring/management, and early exercise/mobility bundle. Crit Care Med 2014;42(5):1024–36.
34. Hsieh SJ, Otusanya O, Gershengorn HB, et al. Staged implementation of awakening and breathing, coordination, delirium monitoring and management, and early mobilization bundle improves patient outcomes and reduces hospital costs. Crit Care Med 2019;47(7):885–93.
35. Pun BT, Balas MC, Barnes-Daly MA, et al. Caring for critically ill patients with the ABCDEF bundle: results of the ICU liberation collaborative in over 15,000 adults. Crit Care Med 2019;47(1):3–14.
36. Rhodes A, Evans LE, Alhazzani W, et al. Surviving sepsis campaign: international guidelines for management of sepsis and septic shock: 2016. Intensive Care Med 2017;43(3):304–77.
37. Donovan AL, Aldrich JM, Gross AK, et al. Interprofessional care and teamwork in the ICU. Crit Care Med 2018;46(6):980–90.
38. James FR, Power N, Laha S. Decision-making in intensive care medicine - a review. J Intensive Care Soc 2018;19(3):247–58.
39. Lundgren-Laine H, Kontio E, Perttila J, et al. Managing daily intensive care activities: an observational study concerning ad hoc decision making of charge nurses and intensivists. Crit Care 2011;15(4):R188.
40. Jones D, DeVita M, Warrillow S. Ten clinical indicators suggesting the need for ICU admission after Rapid Response Team review. Intensive Care Med 2016;42(2):261–3.
41. Blanch L, Abillama FF, Amin P, et al. Triage decisions for ICU admission: report from the Task Force of the World Federation of Societies of intensive and critical care medicine. J Crit Care 2016;36:301–5.

42. Sprung CL, Danis M, Iapichino G, et al. Triage of intensive care patients: identifying agreement and controversy. Intensive Care Med 2013;39(11):1916–24.

43. Chalfin DB. Denied and delayed care: the synergy between the emergency department and the ICU. Crit Care Med 2018;46(5):814–5.

44. Dichter JR, Devereaux A. Leadership during a disaster. In: Farmer JC, Wax RS, Baldisseri MR, editors. Preparing your ICU for disaster response. 1st edition. Chicago: Society of Critical Care; 2012. p. 23–48.

45. Singh JM, MacDonald RD. Pro/con debate: do the benefits of regionalized critical care delivery outweigh the risks of interfacility patient transport? Crit Care 2009; 13(4):219.

46. Singh JM, MacDonald RD, Ahghari M. Critical events during land-based interfacility transport. Ann Emerg Med 2014;64(1):9–15.e12.

47. Kupas DF, Wang HE. Critical care paramedics—a missing component for safe interfacility transport in the United States. Ann Emerg Med 2014;64(1):17–8.

48. Odetola FO, Davis MM, Cohn LM, et al. Interhospital transfer of critically ill and injured children: an evaluation of transfer patterns, resource utilization, and clinical outcomes. J Hosp Med 2009;4(3):164–70.

49. King MA, Niven AS, Beninati W, et al. Evacuation of the ICU: care of the critically ill and injured during pandemics and disasters: CHEST consensus statement. Chest 2014;146(4 Suppl):e44S–60S.

50. Rozenfeld RA, Reynolds SL, Ewing S, et al. Development of an evacuation tool to facilitate disaster preparedness: use in a planned evacuation to support a hospital move. Disaster Med Public Health Prep 2017;11(4):479–86.

51. Janz DR, Khan YA, Mooney JL, et al. Effect of interhospital ICU relocation on patient physiology and clinical outcomes. J Intensive Care Med 2017. [Epub ahead of print].

52. Hick JL, Hanfling D, Cantrill SV. Allocating scarce resources in disasters: emergency department principles. Ann Emerg Med 2012;59(3):177–87.

53. Uppal A, Evans L, Chitkara N, et al. In search of the silver lining: the impact of Superstorm Sandy on Bellevue Hospital. Ann Am Thorac Soc 2013;10(2):135–42.

Preparing the Intensive Care Unit for Disaster

Randy S. Wax, MD, MEd, FRCPC, FCCM

KEYWORDS

- Disaster • Emergency preparedness • Disaster preparedness • Critical care
- Intensive care • Hazard-vulnerability analysis • Disaster exercise
- Disaster simulation

KEY POINTS

- Critical care disaster preparedness should balance all-hazards versus hazard-specific approaches. A critical care-specific hazard-vulnerability analysis can be conducted to identify priorities for hazard-specific planning.
- When a critical care team prepares for disaster, the entire interprofessional team should have an opportunity for input. Broad stakeholder input from other services within the hospital should also be sought, especially when planning for special populations, such as pediatric and obstetric critically ill patients.
- Critical care teams should regularly participate in disaster exercises to test and refine their plans based on immediate and delayed reflective feedback. Focus should include practice of unfamiliar tasks (eg, hospital incident command system, disaster triage, biohazard infection control) and use of disaster-specific equipment (eg, advanced personal protective equipment, stockpile mechanical ventilators).

There are 4 phases of disaster management: mitigation, preparedness, response, and recovery. This article focuses on critical care preparedness aspects of disaster management by discussing what disaster scenarios should be considered, who should be involved in disaster preparedness, and some recommendations for preparedness efforts. Effective preparedness will increase the effectiveness of disaster mitigation, disaster response, and disaster recovery. Unfortunately, interest in disaster preparedness waxes and wanes depending on the temporal proximity of the latest disaster threat, and often focuses efforts on the last disaster instead of the next one.[1]

FOR WHAT DISASTER SHOULD WE PREPARE?

Disaster preparedness must strike a balance between all-hazards and hazard-specific approaches. The all-hazards approach takes into account generic threats to critical care demand and supply issues regardless of the cause of the disaster or surge event.

Disclosure: The author has no conflict of interest to disclose.
Department of Critical Care Medicine, Lakeridge Health, Lakeridge/Durham Clinical Hub, Queen's University, 1 Hospital Court, Oshawa, Ontario L1G 2B9, Canada
E-mail address: randy.wax@queensu.ca

The hazard-specific approach creates a plan that is tailored to a specific type of event. Advantages and disadvantages of both approaches are summarized in **Table 1**. An all-hazards approach has the advantage of being potentially applicable to all possible events; however, it may create a less effective response due to lack of planning for specific challenges (eg, dialysis resources for crush injury-related renal failure after a major earthquake). A hazard-specific approach works well for the disaster events considered during planning; however, an unexpected type of event may result in a challenging response in the early stages of the disaster until the response can be recalibrated.[2]

Disaster preparedness efforts should include a hazard-vulnerability analysis (HVA), which evaluates risk by taking into account the likelihood of an event occurring, the severity of impact should such an event occur, the current state of preparedness, and internal/external capability to respond (RISK = PROBABILITY $\times$ SEVERITY). For health care organizations, the Kaiser Permanente model provides an excellent example of such a framework and provides some online tools (such as their Hazard and Vulnerability Assessment Tool) to help hospitals prepare an HVA.[3] Generating risk scores or rankings for different types of disaster events can help prioritize preparedness efforts by focusing on the most likely or most severe types of events, keeping in mind the need to maintain some level of all-hazards preparedness in case the HVA proves inaccurate or that a highly unlikely event occurs.

An HVA may be conducted from different perspectives, with different results. Federal, state/province, county/region, and local hospitals may note different probabilities, potential impact, and levels of preparedness creating different risk profiles. For example, a nuclear power plant disaster may be much less likely than natural disasters from a federal or state perspective; however, a hospital system located in close proximity to 2 nuclear power plants (such as the one in which this author practices) should likely take such events much more seriously in their planning efforts.

Even within a hospital, the results of an HVA may be more or less generalizable to different areas/programs within the hospital. The emergency department (ED) and operating room would typically experience a huge impact in a sudden onset trauma surge (such as a mass casualty shooting), whereas a bioterrorism or pandemic event with a prolonged incubation period may have a greater effect on the intensive care unit (ICU) because of the prolonged need for mechanical ventilation and ICU support for disaster-related patients. Hence the importance of involving critical care in

Table 1
Characteristics of all-hazards versus hazard-specific approaches to disaster preparedness

All-Hazards approach	Hazard-Specific approach
Harder to prepare because of lack of specific threat	Easier to prepare response to known threat
Onset, duration, and scale of event unclear	Onset, duration, and scale of event understood during planning
Cannot address specific incident-related concerns in advance	Specific incident-related concerns can be addressed
Requires a dynamic response with recalibration to meet the needs of a specific event	Fixed response to specific event, but may require ongoing recalibration of a minor nature
Prepared for initial response regardless of type of disaster	Specific hazard may not occur despite prioritization through hazard-vulnerability analysis

hospital-wide disaster planning, but also ensuring that the critical care team conducts independent disaster preparedness activities to consider issues specific to the ICU.

WHO SHOULD BE INVOLVED IN HOSPITAL CRITICAL CARE DISASTER PLANNING AND HOW CAN THEY CONTRIBUTE?

Given that critical care is by nature an interprofessional health care effort, the need for interprofessional involvement in critical care disaster planning should be obvious. Understanding the potential roles for usual members of the critical care team in disaster planning should help guide expectations and accountabilities in the planning process. In addition, clarity of the nature of the ideal 2-way interaction with noncritical care stakeholders inside and outside the hospital is essential, thus encouraging the sharing of critical care expertise with others to help with their planning efforts and improving critical care planning with expert internal input. **Table 2** highlights potential contributions of different stakeholders toward critical care disaster planning, with further details discussed below.

Critical Care Physicians

Critical care physicians possess key understanding of the nature of organ failure and support, and have day-to-day experience with patient prioritization and triage activities. Strong critical care physician presence and leadership in disaster planning is essential for developing an adequate and sustainable critical care physician resource plan for disaster events.[4] As part of disaster planning, critical care physicians can help design an education strategy to prepare noncritical care physicians to assist in a disaster event as ICU physician extenders, often deployed using a just-in-time approach at the time of a disaster. Critical care physicians can also work with physicians in other areas of the hospital likely to provide critical care outside the ICU during a disaster, such as the ED, to ensure their planning takes into account critical care capacity.

Critical Care Nursing and Other Providers

As essential frontline care providers for any critically ill patient, critical care nursing must be involved in ICU disaster planning.[5] Key factors for consideration include appropriate and sustainable nursing staffing (including potentially modified nurse:patient ratios), modifications to care standards if required, and documentation requirements. Planning for use of ICU nursing extenders with non-ICU nurses requires advance clarification of the scope of non-ICU nurses in caring for critically ill patients and creation of just-in-time education support to allow non-ICU nurses to augment their ability to contribute during a disaster. Critical care nursing leadership involvement will ensure adequate planning for the required interfaces between the ICU and other areas of the hospital from a patient safety and administrative perspective, including strategies for bed management and patient flow into and out of the ICU.

Advanced nursing providers, such as nurse practitioners and nurse anesthetists,[6] and other providers, such as physician assistants and critical care paramedics, may provide helpful input during the planning process. In particular, these providers can help others understand how leveraging their enhanced scopes of practice may provide additional support during a severe critical care surge.

Respiratory Therapists

Respiratory therapist expertise is required to ensure appropriate planning for availability of medical gas (especially oxygen) in ICU and non-ICU clinical spaces, adequate

Table 2
Highlights of potential contributions from different stakeholders during critical care disaster preparedness efforts

Stakeholder	Potential Contributions to Critical Care Disaster Planning
Critical care physicians	• Develop physician resource plan, including strategies to train and integrate non-ICU physicians into the surged ICU patient care team • Determine procedures for assisting other areas of the hospital (eg, emergency department) during early phases of a disaster before the wave of patients being received by the ICU
Critical care nursing, advanced practice nurses (nurse practitioners, nurse anesthetists), physician assistants, critical care paramedics	• Develop staffing strategies, including integration of non-ICU nursing support into surged ICU patient care team • Identify opportunities to maximize scope of practice and contribution from advanced providers
Respiratory therapists	• Planning for medical gas and ventilatory support equipment, including in nontraditional care areas to manage critically ill patients • Education and practice with nonfamiliar stockpile ventilators
Pharmacists	• Provide advice on appropriate medications to stockpile for all-hazards and hazard-specific plans
Dieticians, physiotherapists, and occupational therapists	• Develop mitigation strategies to maintain adequate nutrition and rehabilitation during surge demand for services • Create just-in-time educational tools to help family members assist with rehabilitation activities
Mental health clinicians, social workers, chaplaincy, and clinical ethicists	• Develop plan for advance stress inoculation for hospital staff • Plan for need to support patients, family members, and hospital staff during and after a disaster
Trauma, emergency department, and perioperative services	• Develop plans for mutual assistance between programs tailored to different phases of a disaster, including need for suspension of elective surgical activity • Ensure mechanisms for transfer of accountability are in place despite surge in patient mobility
Pediatric, neonatal, and obstetric services	• Determine specific equipment and supply needs to support these special patient populations • Anticipate need to support pediatric critical care in nonpediatric hospitals during a disaster event
Laboratory and diagnostic imaging services	• Plan for enhanced point-of-care testing/studies to expedite clinical decision making and reduce demand on overwhelmed staff
Facilities and information technology	• Prepare for modifications to create more negative-pressure airborne isolation space • Ensure adequate and flexible network coverage to allow use of mobile computers in makeshift clinical areas
Security	• Anticipate access control needs for traditional and makeshift critical care clinical areas

(continued on next page)

Table 2 (continued)	
Stakeholder	Potential Contributions to Critical Care Disaster Planning
	• Provide support for staff during challenging interactions with family members, particularly during communication of triage decisions
Administration and finance	• Provide support for critical care disaster preparedness activities • Secure external funding when possible to offset the costs of disaster preparedness (eg, medication and equipment stockpiles, staff education)

access to airway equipment and mechanical ventilators, and planning for provision of respiratory support in non-ICU areas of the hospital.[7] Strategies for enhancing capacity for mechanical ventilation may rely on use of unfamiliar ventilators from an external stockpile, or use of modified ventilators (such as transport ventilators or anesthesia gas machines). Respiratory therapists may also help with other aspects of hazard-specific preparedness, such as strategies for monitoring of carbon monoxide in mass casualty exposures or delivery of bronchodilators for patients exposed to pulmonary irritants. In many jurisdictions, respiratory therapists with maximized scope of practice can also provide support for nonrespiratory issues, such as intravenous insertion or medication delivery, that can be incorporated into planning for provider oversight of patients during a major surge event.

Pharmacists

Appropriate stockpiling of medications is an essential component of critical care disaster preparedness, for which pharmacist input is invaluable.[8] From an all-hazards perspective, generic medication requirements for management of ICU patients can be modeled, such as need for sedation and analgesia for ventilated patients, or preventative therapy such as deep venous thrombosis prophylaxis. Hazard-specific planning can include medications specific to address the hazard, such as antidotes for organophosphate poisoning, cyanide exposure treatment, or antiviral medications for pandemic influenza. The ICU-specific HVA can help pharmacists prioritize medication planning during disaster preparedness activities. Knowledge of factors such as shelf life of medications, need for special storage such as refrigeration, and costing helps pharmacists provide essential advice for procurement. Ideally, stockpiling strategies will avoid unnecessary availability of multiple drugs that can provide the same effect, such as having morphine and fentanyl and hydromorphone available as multiple narcotics. Pharmacy input for creation of preprinted order sets to be used during a disaster can help align prescribing by providers with the available drugs stockpiled. Finally, given that funds used for disaster preparedness take away from funds required for usual hospital expenses, pharmacy input on cost:benefit ratios of different medication options can help with a fiscally responsible approach to disaster planning and logistics.

Dieticians, Physiotherapists, and Occupational Therapists

Maintaining appropriate nutrition, early mobilization, and encouraging improved recovery to baseline functional state are essential adjuncts to life-support efforts. Encouraging the involvement of relevant interprofessional team members in critical care disaster planning can help determine potential limitations in services during a disaster, suggest mitigation strategies to minimize the impact of a surge in demand for their expertise, and propose educational strategies to use other health care staff and even family members to assist as extenders with less frequent available input from these health care professionals.

Mental Health Clinicians, Social Workers, Chaplaincy, and Clinical Ethicists

Critical care disaster planning should take into account the tremendous stress of such events on patients, families and clinical staff. More detailed discussion of these issues can be found in other articles in this issue. Although prehospital and ED triage strategies should identify and support disaster victims with isolated psychological/mental health issues, nothing precludes the copresence of mental health injuries (novel or exacerbations of existing mental health diagnoses) with critical illness from physical causes. Planning for availability of psychiatry and other mental health consultation-liaison services should be considered to support patients requiring critical care after a disaster. Similarly, family members of critically ill patients will require ongoing support throughout the hospitalization of their loved ones, which may include need for social work and chaplaincy. Strategies to ensure effective communication and support of family members when patients require transfer out of the hospital for higher level of care or capacity reasons should be considered in planning efforts. Withdrawal of active life support may be required when patients are not benefiting from critical care support and/or if triage decision making requires shifting of resources to patients more likely to benefit, and the involvement of clinical ethicists to support patients, families, and staff members can be very helpful thus requiring consideration during planning.[9] An emerging concept in disaster planning incorporates the concept of mental health/stress inoculation for hospital staff, which may include advance and just-in-time deployment to increase performance during the disaster and prevent long-term psychological effects.[10,11]

Trauma, Emergency Department, and Perioperative Services

During events that cause a sudden and rapid surge of patients to the hospital with mass casualty medical issues, trauma/burns, or other injuries requiring surgical support, impact on the ICU can be delayed but substantial as the disaster unfolds. In such circumstances, the ED is usually on the frontline as first receivers of critically ill patients. The ED and ICU teams must collaborate during disaster planning to ensure that critically ill patients receive optimal care regardless of their geographic location within the hospital. In the early stages of a disaster, ICU planning may need to include a time-limited option to have critical care clinicians support patient care and triage activities in the ED. Many patients will require resuscitation and stabilization in the ED before being safe to transport to the ICU, and may also require transfer to the operating room for damage control or definitive surgery before transfer to the ICU. Planning for the orderly and safe transfer of patients from the ED or the operating room to the ICU should include strategies for efficient transfer of clinical information and accountability of care.

In the event of a nonsurgical disaster creating severe patient surge within the ICU and hospital as a whole, disaster planning should include procedures for decision making regarding the cancellation of elective surgery to augment availability of space, staff and, supplies for disaster-related patients.[12] Plans for using surgical resources to support critically ill patients in the postoperative recovery room area (as an extended ICU) or operating rooms (using anesthetic gas machine ventilators) should be discussed collaboratively.

Pediatrics, Neonatal, and Obstetric Services

Pediatric specialty hospitals that have a distinct pediatric critical care unit often provide regional support for critically ill and injured children. In a disaster event, the dedicated pediatric critical care center may be overwhelmed with patients, or the nature of the disaster may preclude immediate transfer of pediatric patients. Therefore, nonpediatric hospitals should plan for management of pediatric patients. This would require potential stockpiling of equipment and supplies appropriate for pediatric patients. Advance or just-in-time education for nonpediatric critical care providers to manage critically ill children should be considered (1 course currently recommended for this purpose in some jurisdictions is the Pediatric Fundamental Critical Care Support Course offered by the Society of Critical Care Medicine[13,14]), as well as planned partnership with pediatricians to comanage critically ill children with adult intensivists.

A disaster may force hospitals to care for obstetric patients beyond their usual complexity case mix or with gestational age earlier than usual, resulting in neonatal patients requiring more support than usually provided at the facility. These patients may have issues related to the disaster, or may be unable to be transferred because of the overwhelming surge in the usual tertiary care facility or because of the disrupted patient transport resources. From a critical care perspective, collaboration with obstetric teams will be required for management of critically ill pregnant patients. Neonatal ICUs may need to work with adult critical care teams to gain access to additional neonatal-capable mechanical ventilators and monitoring equipment for their patients, or may face requests to share their ventilators to support an adult critical care surge.

For these special groups of potentially critically ill patients, the critical care team and hospital at large should take account of space, equipment, supplies, and staff to help manage surges for those groups. In the absence of expertise to manage these patient populations, hospitals should consider planning to leverage telemedicine technology[15–17] to gain assistance from clinical experts at a remote site (which may be different than their usual partners who may be also affected by the disaster and unable to assist).

Laboratory and Diagnostic Imaging Services

From an all-hazards perspective, a disaster can change the need for laboratory and diagnostic imaging support because of the increased demand for tests and the need for rapid, point-of-care results to minimize delay in clinical decision making and triage decisions during mass casualty events. From a laboratory perspective, disaster planning should incorporate strategies for triaging of laboratory study requests to maximize time-sensitive results impacting on critical clinical decision making. Use of existing or stockpiled portable point-of-care laboratory equipment that can be operated by frontline clinical staff can be considered to reduce burden on the laboratory team. Bedside clinical monitoring may be used as a laboratory test mitigation strategy in some cases, such as the use of pulse oximetry and quantitative capnography for ventilated patients instead of arterial blood gas testing, or advanced pulse oximeters that can measure carbon monoxide levels as a screening strategy in mass casualty carbon monoxide exposure.[18] Certain high-priority threats identified by the ICU-specific HVA may warrant specific discussion with laboratory services to ensure availability of necessary hazard-specific testing if possible. Blood bank services in particular will need to coordinate with critical care and other hospital services to prepare for mass casualty events placing excessive demands for blood products, including a strategy to triage blood product requests in extreme cases.

During a disaster, demand for diagnostic imaging studies may outstrip capacity of available equipment and technologists, and availability of radiologists to interpret the studies. Use of portable radiographic equipment with an integrated monitor to allow immediate review of images by frontline clinicians may reduce delay in detection of critical clinically important findings. Planning for enhanced availability of point-of-care ultrasound can be helpful as a substitute for other diagnostic imaging modalities, or to help triage cases when resources are limited, such as prioritizing computed tomography scan requests for possible abdominal injuries or ruling out of a pneumothorax and avoiding need for portable radiographic equipment.[19] Other newer point-of-care technology may help identify patients at higher risk for neurosurgical intervention and again help prioritize patients for access to limited diagnostic resources.[20]

Facilities and Information Technology

An essential element of critical care disaster planning assumes the high likelihood of having to manage critically ill patients outside of the usual ICU space. Ensuring that appropriate physical plant and space is available, along with information technology support, will reduce some challenges with regard to working in non-ICU space. Understanding of space capabilities, with the input of facilities engineers, can help with the appropriate planning choices for ICU surge space within the hospital and help avoid unpleasant surprises, such as lack of emergency backup power outlets, sufficient medical gas supply, or other limitations. A particular concern is the availability of negative-pressure airborne isolation rooms in the event of a serious airborne-spread biohazard disaster. Most hospitals have limited airborne isolation capacity during usual operations. During hospital surge experiences during the worldwide 2012 to 2013 Severe Acute Respiratory Syndrome (SARS) outbreak, some facilities were able to modify airflow and erect barriers to create large negative-pressure isolation wards, including ICUs.[21] Planning for various scenarios identified in the ICU-specific HVA should identify potential physical facility gaps and prompt mitigation strategies.

Intensive care units are technology-dependent areas of care that rely on sophisticated information technology services for networking of patient care monitors and equipment, electronic drug dispensing modules, and computer access to support ICU-specific electronic medical records. In disaster situations, initial receipt of patients in the ED will often shift to a paper-based triage and registration strategy. Planning for the transition from the initial crisis phase of a disaster with mass casualties to integration of patients within the electronic medical record will help ensure timely and accurate access and creation of health provider notes, laboratory results, and diagnostic imaging reports. Information technology services should also plan for additional need of mobile computers and sufficient wireless network access to manage critically ill patients outside of the usual ICU space. The potential need for use of telemedicine services to support management of special populations of patients, as mentioned above, should prompt planning and testing of telemedicine capacity including equipment and network bandwidth in advance to prevent service gaps during a disaster.

Security

Hospitals typically spend considerable effort and resources on controlling external access to the facility during disaster events to ensure patient and staff safety, deter premature entry of persons requiring decontamination, maintain control of limited resources and supplies, and prevent unauthorized members of the media or other members of the public from compromising patient and family privacy.[22] In the event of strict hospital visitor restrictions, attempts to circumvent security controls can be expected. Specific consideration of the security needs of the critical care areas (traditional and makeshift) is occasionally overlooked. Intense emotional reactions of family and friends of critically ill patients can occur and be compounded in a stressful disaster situation. In the event of implementation of triage activities and a shift from usual standards of care, decisions to withdraw life support from those patients not benefiting from scarce resources can be met with violent objection. Physical measures to limit access to the critical care areas may need enhancement, and there may also be a need for greater visible presence of security staff as a deterrent to unacceptable treatment of hospital staff. Liaison with security staff should be included as part of the critical care disaster planning process to avoid gaps in security capability.

Administration and Finance

Disaster preparedness requires an investment of resources in terms of staff time to commit to planning, equipment, and supplies earmarked for disaster stockpiling, and development of relationships and agreements with external entities. For preparedness to be effective, hospital administration must appreciate the need for planning and endorse recommendations. Although the finance elements within a hospital are usually prepared to capture costs incurred while a disaster is in progress to facilitate reimbursement, advance efforts to secure funding support for disaster preparedness through government and other agency grants can mitigate opposition to diversion of funds away from frontline clinical activities. Increasingly, hospitals are appointing a lead for disaster preparedness who can act as a liaison between clinicians and administration. Given the high costs that can be associated with provision of critical care, particularly in surge situations, clear articulation of the needs for critical care disaster planning may enable the necessary allocation of resources to ensure the planning vision is realized.

HOW CAN WE TEACH, TEST, AND TWEAK THE CRITICAL CARE DISASTER PLAN?

Certainly, lessons can be learned after each disaster event that can lead to identification of problems or gaps in a critical care disaster plan. Fortunately, those disaster events are uncommon, but, unfortunately, we cannot rely only on actual disaster events to test plans and maintain disaster competency among hospital staff. Frequent disaster exercises can help educate staff on how to function during an actual event, and provide feedback to disaster planners allowing plan improvement before a disaster. Disaster exercises may vary in scale and fidelity (**Fig. 1**). The scale of a disaster exercise may be limited to a single critical care unit, involve multiple hospital services, or be expanded to a regional, state, or even national scale. The fidelity of a disaster exercise may be tabletop-based, using patient cards and virtual clinical spaces; may take into account current actual clinical volumes and bed availability; or may use hundreds of actors playing the role of patients, combined with high-fidelity patient simulators, scattered throughout actual areas of the hospital for an in-situ exercise.[23] Exercises of greater fidelity and greater scale consume more resources to conduct, and may be more likely to interfere with routine hospital operations. However, the greater the fidelity and the greater the scale, the more likely it will be to identify opportunities for improvement in disaster planning. Thus, a balance of these factors must take into account local resources, support for disaster preparedness by hospital leadership, and mandatory activities required for hospital accreditation or government funding.

Beyond generic disaster exercise activities, certain aspects of disaster planning specific to critical care should be specifically addressed in exercise design. Critical care leaders and staff should understand the Hospital Incident Command System (HICS)[24]

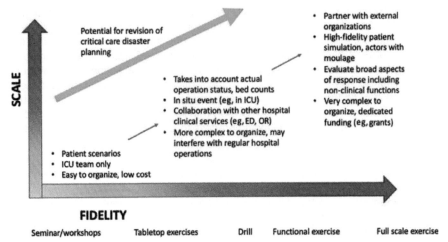

Fig. 1. Design of critical care disaster exercises taking into account scale and fidelity of planned events.

as organized in their hospital, and know how they interface with the HICS. Critical care would normally fit within the Operations branch, under control of the Operations Chief. In some cases, leadership roles within the HICS may be filled by critical care leaders given their broad clinical understanding of the hospital as a whole; however, their responsibilities would be guided by the HICS role rather than keeping a narrow focus on critical care. Depending on the nature of the disaster event, critical care leaders and clinicians may be asked to assist the HICS leadership team as subject matter experts, or participate in task forces or strike groups designed to handle specific problems. Certain principles of the HICS can be useful in disaster planning on a smaller scale specific to critical care. The concept of span of control, having everyone report to only 1 person, and each person only having 5 to 7 people reporting to them, may be helpful in organizing clinical teams including non-ICU staff supervised by ICU clinicians. Also, the concept of job action sheets that provide guidance for key actions given a particular role can be helpful in reminding staff of key tasks during a stressful disaster event, and can be a valuable teaching tool during an exercise.

Hospital exercises often emphasize infrequent but important tasks, such as decontamination of patients before entry to hospital, which are important but potentially less relevant to critical care staff. Patients should never enter a critical care area without decontamination if required. For biological infectious events, there may be no ability to perform the equivalent of decontamination, because the patients remain infectious and put staff and other patients at risk. Exercise and evaluation of advanced infection control strategies (such as conversion to negative-pressure clinical areas, use of infection control coaches), or advanced personal protective equipment (such as powered air-purifying respirator use, safe donning and doffing of equipment) may be of special significance for critical care team preparedness. Exercises should also encourage familiarity with stockpile equipment, such as monitoring equipment or unfamiliar ventilators, so that there is some retention of competency in the event of the need to use such equipment in a disaster event. Just-in-time education strategies to augment clinical care for special populations (eg, pediatrics) or hazard-specific care (eg, radiation sickness) can be practiced and evaluated for future revision.

Much of the learning from a disaster exercise takes place during the debriefing phases after the event. A "hotwash" debriefing immediately after the event can capture important lessons; however, another opportunity to capture additional lessons after some time to reflect can also provide further guidance on disaster plan revisions. Preparing an after-action report after simulated and real disasters can ensure that lessons learned are captured; however, development of a list of actions including accountabilities and timelines, with a process for follow-up to ensure completion, should reduce the rediscovery of the same recommendations at the next real or simulated disaster.

SUMMARY

The preparedness phase of disaster management can make or break the response to an actual disaster. Teams should aim for an optimal balance between flexible all-hazards preparedness and hazard-specific preparedness guided by the hazard-vulnerability assessment. One of the best strategies for ensuring ongoing support for disaster preparedness activities is to identify potential flaws in the current disaster plan through frequent disaster exercises. Despite the temptation to divert resources to routine clinical budget demands, an upfront investment in preparedness will hopefully lead to a more efficient disaster response and more rapid recovery to normal operations should a disaster occur.

REFERENCES

1. Kollek D, Jarvis C. Disaster preparedness: are we ready yet? Hospital News 2019. Available at: https://hospitalnews.com/33869-2/. Accessed June 16, 2019.
2. Gregory AP. Reassessing the effectiveness of all-hazards planning in emergency management. Inquiries Journal 2015. Available at: http://www.inquiriesjournal.com/articles/1050/reassessing-the-effectiveness-of-all-hazards-planning-in-emergency-management. Accessed June 16, 2019.
3. Hazards vulnerability analysis. Emergency preparedness: California Hospital Association. Available at: https://www.calhospitalprepare.org/hazard-vulnerability-analysis. Accessed June 16, 2019.
4. Shirley PJ, Mandersloot G. Clinical review: the role of the intensive care physician in mass casualty incidents: planning, organisation, and leadership. Crit Care 2008;12(3):214.
5. Loke AY, Fung OW. Nurses' competencies in disaster nursing: implications for curriculum development and public health. Int J Environ Res Public Health 2014;11(3):3289–303.
6. American Association of Nurse Anesthetists. Guidelines regarding the role of the certified registered nurse anesthetist in mass casualty incident preparedness and response. 2014. Available at: https://www.aana.com/docs/default-source/practice-aana-com-web-documents-(all)/guidelines-regarding-the-role-of-the-crna-in-mass-casualty-incident-preparedness-and-response.pdf?sfvrsn=870049b1_4. Accessed June 16, 2019.
7. Laberge ML. Creating a disaster plan for RT departments. Can J Respir Ther 2017;53(2):42–3.
8. Bell C, Daniel S. Pharmacy Leader's role in hospital emergency preparedness planning. Hosp Pharm 2014;49(4):398–404.
9. Biddison LD, Berkowitz KA, Courtney B, et al. Ethical considerations: care of the critically ill and injured during pandemics and disasters: CHEST consensus statement. Chest 2014;146(4 Suppl):e145S-55S.

10. Maunder RG, Lancee WJ, Mae R, et al. Computer-assisted resilience training to prepare healthcare workers for pandemic influenza: a randomized trial of the optimal dose of training. BMC Health Serv Res 2010;10:72.
11. Aiello A, Khayeri MY, Raja S, et al. Resilience training for hospital workers in anticipation of an influenza pandemic. J Contin Educ Health Prof 2011;31(1):15–20.
12. American Society of Anesthesiologists Committee on Trauma and Emergency Preparedness. Emergency preparedness: manual for anesthesia department organization and management. Available at: https://www.asahq.org/~/media/sites/asahq/files/public/resources/asa%20committees/madom%20emergency%20preparedness%20chapter-final.pdf. Accessed June 16, 2019.
13. Western New York Pediatric Surge Work Group. WNY hospital pediatric disaster preparedness presentation 2014-15. Available at: https://www.urmc.rochester.edu/MediaLibraries/URMCMedia/flrtc/documents/WNY-Pediatric-WG-Planning-Steps-for-Hospitals-2014-15_2.ppt. Accessed June 16, 2019.
14. New York City Pediatric Disaster Coalition and New York City Department of Health and Mental Hygiene. Recommendations for increasing NYC pediatric critical care surge capacity (Draft). 2009. Available at: https://www.urmc.rochester.edu/MediaLibraries/URMCMedia/flrtc/documents/hepp-pedsconf02-rec-for-incr-picu-surge.pdf. Accessed June 16, 2019.
15. Harvey JB, Yeager BE, Cramer C, et al. The impact of telemedicine on pediatric critical care triage. Pediatr Crit Care Med 2017;18(11):e555–60.
16. Ellenby MS, Marcin JP. The role of telemedicine in pediatric critical care. Crit Care Clin 2015;31(2):275–90.
17. Sauers-Ford HS, Marcin JP, Underwood MA, et al. The use of telemedicine to address disparities in access to specialist care for neonates. Telemed J E Health 2018. https://doi.org/10.1089/tmj.2018.0095.
18. Sebbane M, Claret PG, Mercier G, et al. Emergency department management of suspected carbon monoxide poisoning: role of pulse CO-oximetry. Respir Care 2013;58(10):1614–20.
19. Alrajhi K, Woo MY, Vaillancourt C. Test characteristics of ultrasonography for the detection of pneumothorax: a systematic review and meta-analysis. Chest 2012; 141(3):703–8.
20. Leon-Carrion J, Dominguez-Roldan JM, Leon-Dominguez U, et al. The Infrascanner, a handheld device for screening in situ for the presence of brain haematomas. Brain Inj 2010;24(10):1193–201.
21. Loutfy MR, Wallington T, Rutledge T, et al. Hospital preparedness and SARS. Emerg Infect Dis 2004;10(5):771–6.
22. Sarr E, McGlen K. Lessons healthcare security professionals learned from Hurricane Harvey. Security Management. Alexandria (VA): ASIS International; 2019. Available at: https://sm.asisonline.org/Pages/Lessons-Healthcare-Security-Professionals-Learned-from-Hurricane-Harvey.aspx. Accessed June 16, 2019.
23. World Health Organization. Hospital and health facility emergency exercises: guidance materials. 2010. Available at: http://www.wpro.who.int/publications/docs/HospitalandHealthFacilityEmergencyExercisesforWeb.pdf. Accessed June 16, 2019.
24. Emergency Medical Services Authority California. Hospital incident command system guidebook. 5th edition 2014. Available at: https://emsa.ca.gov/wp-content/uploads/sites/71/2017/09/HICS_Guidebook_2014_11.pdf. Accessed June 16, 2019.

Augmenting Critical Care Capacity in a Disaster

Gilbert Seda, MD, PhD*, John S. Parrish, MD

KEYWORDS

- Disaster response • Surge capacity • Augmentation • Mass critical care
- Tele-critical care • Virtual critical care

KEY POINTS

- Surge capacity in mass critical care refers to an intensive care unit's ability to rapidly expand care to as many patients as possible in a disaster.
- The 4 necessary components of surge capacity are staff, supplies, space, and structure.
- Augmentation of critical care staff involves utilization of noncritical care staff with oversight by critical care staff.
- Virtual critical care or tele-critical care can augment critical care staff by providing specialized consultation and monitoring.

INTRODUCTION

Staffing of critical care units by intensivists is the standard of care and recommended by the Leapfrog group,[1] the Society of Critical Care Medicine,[2] and the American Academy of Critical Care Medicine.[3] Unfortunately, there is a national shortage of critical care providers and critical care beds in the United States and it will continue to get worse with the aging population. Annually, critical care services in the United States account for $81.7 billion, with most of the care spent on the elderly population.[4] As the percentage of adults older than 65 continues to increase over the next 10 to 20 years, the number of intensivists nationally will be unable to meet current needs.[5] Of US hospitals, 57% reported difficulty filling critical care nursing vacancies in addition to an aging critical care nursing population.[6] In areas with limited critical care resources, tele-critical care, also referred to as virtual critical care, allows hospitals with limited staffing to receive consultation and monitoring by intensivists.[7] The shortage of critical care personnel has detrimental effects on the care of the critically ill, as studies have shown that patient care by intensivists reduces mortality and decreases length of hospital stay.[8,9]

Disclosure Statement: The authors have no disclosures.
Department of Pulmonary and Critical Care Medicine, Naval Medical Center San Diego, 34800 Bob Wilson Drive, Suite 301, San Diego, CA 92134, USA
* Corresponding author.
E-mail address: gilbert.seda@gmail.com

Crit Care Clin 35 (2019) 563–573
https://doi.org/10.1016/j.ccc.2019.06.007
0749-0704/19/Published by Elsevier Inc.

In the event of a disaster, whether it be a nuclear event, pandemic, bioterrorism, earthquake, or mass shooting, successful management requires health care delivery system ability to provide rapid mass critical care services. The first step in providing mass critical care is preparation and training. Hospitals must develop a mass casualty plan that clearly articulates what steps need to be implemented to increase critical care resources to accommodate a large number of patients in an all-hazards scenario. This will require surge capacity, which is defined as a health care delivery system's ability to rapidly accommodate an increased demand for critical care services under extraordinary circumstances.[10] To transition to mass critical care services, the 4 essential components of mass critical care are personnel (physicians, critical care nurses, pharmacists, respiratory therapists), equipment (monitors, infusion devices, medications, mechanical ventilation), space (rooms for patients and equipment), and structure.[11]

PREPARATION

Preparation is the first step for all-hazards approach to disaster. Mass casualty incident planning includes an integrated disaster plan, clear chain of command, hazard vulnerability assessment, surge capacity plan, and triage strategy. Hospitals will need an emergency management committee or department whose function is to facilitate disaster training and annual disaster training exercises.[12] Disaster exercises that can help prepare for mass critical care are a mass casualty exercise, a pandemic exercise, a biological or chemical warfare incident, and a hospital evacuation exercise. With respect to mass critical care training, non–critical care staff would benefit from a basic adult critical care course such as the Fundamental Critical Care Support course or a pediatric course such as the Pediatric Fundamental Critical Care, which are both sponsored by the Society of Critical Care Medicine.[13] These courses provide basic concepts essential for critical care, such as recognizing critical illness, airway management, ventilator management, antimicrobial therapy, management of shock, neurocritical care, and basic management of the trauma patient.

There are also courses on disaster management that are sponsored by various organizations and by the federal government. Examples include the Fundamental Disaster Management Course by Society of Critical Care Medicine,[14] and the Disaster Management and Emergency Preparedness Course by the American College of Surgeons.[15] These courses provide an overview of disaster management for medical professionals relevant for those with and without critical care training; however, the courses do not emphasize clinical critical care preparation. Triage in disasters is different from triage in routine hospital care. In disasters, overtriage of patients who do not warrant critical care results in an unavailability of resources for patients who need critical care services. For mental health professions, training in Critical Incident Stress Debriefing is essential in helping with caregiver stress and the long-term psychological effects of a disaster.[16] With respect to preparing civilian bystanders, an important initiative by the American College of Surgeons is the Stop the Bleed training. Death from bleeding can happen within just 5 to 10 minutes, but if civilian bystanders (often the first people on the scene) as well as emergency responders/law enforcement are equipped with basic tools for stopping the bleeding, lives may be saved.[17]

PERSONNEL

Initially, when a hospital faces a disaster, the first step will be the activation of the hospital's mass casualty plan. This will result in a shift from routine hospital operations to disaster triage and mass critical care, with an overall goal of providing care to save as many lives as possible. This will allow hospitals the ability to mobilize their critical care personnel and resources and take the necessary steps to maximize patient volume for the greatest good. This will involve the operations chief of the hospital incident command center taking steps to mobilize their critical care personnel by activating their recall roster, modifying staff schedules, and canceling staff vacations.[18] Critical care personnel involve a multidisciplinary team of specialists that include physicians, nurse practitioners, critical care nurses, and ancillary staff (eg, pharmacists, nutritionist, respiratory therapists, social workers, and physical therapists).[19] An important necessary step for the increase in critical care staffing is the ability of the hospital to provide safety and security for the additional staff and their families (such as food and shelter for the increased staff and their family, including any pets).

In the event there are not enough critical care staff to provide emergency mass critical care, then it will be necessary for a 2-tiered staff model. In this model, intensivists would provide oversight to nonintensivist clinicians and critical care nurses would oversee non–critical care nurses. The guidelines per the Working Group on Mass Critical Care recommends nonintensivists manage approximately 6 critically ill patients and intensivists oversee 4 nonintensivists.[19] In this model, intensivists would provide management of acute emergencies, such as airway management, and nonintensivists would provide routine medical management. This same 2-tiered model would apply to critical care nurses as well as ancillary critical care staff. If possible, a non–critical care nurse should be assigned to no more than 2 critically ill patients, and up to 3 non–critical care nurses may work in collaboration with 1 critical care nurse. Pharmacists and respiratory therapists can supervise pharmacists and respiratory therapists who do not do usually provide critical care. If the number of critically ill patients becomes too large, this 2-tier staff model may have to be adjusted to accommodate the increased number of patients.[19] Rather than lead to a compromise of care, the benefit of the 2-tiered model creates critical care extenders that will help more patients. The challenge will be to avoid overextending care leading to provision of inadequate critical care services, thus the need to consider the span of control of supervising critical care clinicians.

To standardize care and reduce medical errors, hospitals should develop preprinted order sets and use institutional protocols. These can be used for intensive care unit (ICU) triage; the management of hemorrhagic or ischemic stroke; ICU electrolyte management; pain, agitation, and delirium; massive transfusion; post–cardiac arrest resuscitation; anticoagulation reversal; sepsis protocol; hyperglycemic crisis; deep venous thromboembolism; mechanical ventilation; stress ulcer prophylaxis; and prevention of ventilator associated pneumonia.[19,20] Additional order sets for a specific syndrome in a disaster can be developed.

If additional staff are needed that are not available at the hospital, there are several other options. One option is the emergency credentialing of medical volunteers. A hospital's mass casualty plan should have a provision for the emergency credentialing of additional staff.[21] Hospitals in the area that are not affected by the disaster could assist the hospital in the disaster area. Alternatively, you could also transport patients to neighboring hospitals using their critical care capacity and personnel. Another source of volunteers is from critical care professional societies and the federal government.[19] A limitation of this type of staffing is a delay in arrival and they would have a very limited role in a bioterrorism attack. The National Disaster Medical System (NDMS) has Disaster Medical Assistance Teams that are staffed by medical professionals and para-professionals who can provide care, but these health care teams will usually include few critical care professionals.[22] The NDMS will have the ability to transfer patients to another region of the United States; however, these patients would require critical care transport and this process takes some time. Organizations like the Society of Critical Care Medicine may have critical care volunteers, but it is unclear how many would actually help for any given incident and who would fund the volunteers. Finally, a patient's family members also can provide a caretaker role with appropriate guidance, freeing up health care providers for other tasks.

SUPPLIES

In addition to having adequate critical care staff to provide mass critical care, hospitals planning for mass critical care need to have adequate supplies to support critical interventions and understand the supply chains in a disaster.[23] According to the Working Group on Mass Critical Care, priority should be given to interventions that are deemed by critical care experts to improve survival, do not require extraordinary expensive equipment, and can be implemented without consuming an excessive amount of staff time. The essential supplies for mass critical care include personal protective equipment, basic modes of mechanical ventilation, hemodynamic support, antimicrobial therapy or other disease-specific countermeasures, supplemental oxygen, and prophylactic treatments, such as deep vein thrombosis prophylaxis and elevating the head of the bed.[19,23]

Mortality secondary to failure to provide respiratory support for a patient with acute respiratory failure due to acute respiratory distress syndrome (ARDS), pneumonia secondary to inhalation anthrax, or neuromuscular weakness from exposure to a nerve agent is preventable with mechanical ventilation. Hospitals have a number of devices that provide some form of respiratory support to include hospital ventilators, noninvasive ventilation that provide continuous positive airway pressure (CPAP) and bi-level, high-flow oxygen, anesthesia machines, transport ventilators, and, in the worse-case scenario, manual ventilation using bag-valve masks with endotracheal tubes. In a disaster, the basic modes of mechanical ventilation, such as assist-controlled or pressure-controlled ventilation, are adequate for most patients. It is also important for ventilators to have software and circuits so they can provide suitable respiratory support to pediatric patients of all ages and have alarm systems to notify staff of any problems. It is also important for staff to know the battery life of the ventilator in the event there is limited electricity.

Patients who need some form respiratory support without endotracheal intubation can benefit from high-flow oxygen or noninvasive positive pressure devices such as Bi-level or CPAP. In the event there are not enough mechanical ventilators to treat patients with respiratory failure, manual ventilation could be used. Positive end expiratory pressure valves attached to manual resuscitation bags can improve ability to oxygenate, and pressure manometers may help avoid barotrauma through unmonitored excessive ventilation. Studies have not demonstrated a difference between critically ill patients treated by manual ventilation versus mechanical ventilation.[24] A limitation of manual ventilation is that it requires someone to continuously manually ventilate the patient. If the disaster is due to a contagious agent, the person doing the manual ventilation would be at increased risk of infection. It is recommended that local, regional, and states support the stockpiling of basic mechanical ventilators in the event of a pandemic.[25] The Strategic National Stockpile (SNS) includes portable ventilators that can be deployed by the federal government in the event of a disaster but may take a while to reach hospitals.

Shock is another potentially reversible case of mortality in a disaster. Supplies for hemodynamic support are critical and include blood products, crystalloids, and vasopressors. If the disaster is a mass shooting, then it will be important to implement massive transfusion protocols and hemorrhage control for the treatment of hemorrhagic shock. If the disaster is secondary to an Ebola outbreak resulting in septic shock, the management will be fluid resuscitation and vasopressors and personal protective equipment. Although most ICUs continue to use central venous catheters for delivery of vasopressors, there are some preliminary data that suggest that vasopressors administered with peripheral lines in some patients are feasible and safe. One hospital treated more than 730 patients with vasopressors through peripheral intravenous (IV) lines and reported no tissue injuries, although extravasation of vasopressor into subcutaneous tissue occurred in 19 patients (2%, which were recognized and treated).[26] Availability of extravasation kits including phentolamine to block vasoconstriction of extravasated vasopressor can be considered to mitigate this risk. Another multicenter study comparing critically ill patients with central venous catheters versus peripheral venous catheters found more major complications in the peripheral IV group but none of the differences were life threatening.[27] If peripheral IVs are used, they will require close observation by nursing to prevent extravasation. Insertion of intraosseous needles also can be considered as an alternative to central venous catheter placement; however, these typically require removal within 24 hours of insertion.

Additional supplies that are necessary for mass critical care include personal protective equipment, medications (**Table 1**), airway management equipment, Foley catheters, sequential compression devices, crash carts for advanced cardiac life support, volumetric infusion pumps, electronic patient monitors, and parenteral nutrition. When equipment resources are limited, it will be important to sterilize and safely reuse consumables when possible. The Centers for Disease Control and Prevention maintains the SNS in locations around the United States to provide assistance states in a disaster. The SNS has 12-hour push packs of medications, ventilators, and supplies that can be deployed within 12 hours of notification of need.[28] However, the SNS is not intended to function as a first response but rather a resupply for state and local hospitals.

In summary, the CHEST Consensus Statement on surge capacity logistics recommends that mass critical care supplies are interoperable and compatible at regional and state levels to ensure uniformity among facilities. They recommend that facilities have caches of disaster supplies, adequate supply chain resources, and adequate supplies for unique populations to include pediatric, burn, and trauma patients.[29]

Oxygen is a critical consumable resource in mass critical care. The hospital's oxygen supply as well as the supply chain for supplemental oxygen is critical for management of patients with hypoxemia. Hospitals have large quantities of liquid oxygen onsite that is the primary source of wall oxygen supplied to patients. Hospitals typically have redundant systems that are designed to provide a back-up system in the event that one system fails. These systems are efficient and are the safest way to distribute and transport oxygen. These liquid oxygen systems also have alarms in place that notify the hospital when the oxygen needs to be replenished. The alternate source of oxygen is in the form of compressed gas cylinders; however, a strategy would be required to ultimately refill the cylinders. There are 2 types: H cylinders are the large tanks that contain approximately 6900 L of oxygen, and the E cylinders contain approximately 679 L of oxygen. In the event of mass critical care, oxygen cylinders can be used in place of liquid oxygen, but there are safety concerns, as these cylinders are filled to pressures of 2000 to 2200 psi. It is important to know that the SNS does not stockpile oxygen but instead contracts with private vendors to deliver oxygen.[30] In the event of a disaster, these vendors may not be available to the disaster site.

Because oxygen is a critical resource that is often limited in a disaster, proper utilization of supplemental oxygen is important. The British Thoracic Societies Guidelines

Table 1
Medications in emergency mass critical care

Organ System	Drug Class	Medication	Reason for Inclusion in Essential Elements of Critical Care
Neurologic	Sedation and analgesia	Benzodiazepine Opioid Succinylcholine Nondepolarizing paralytic agent	1. Analgesia, anxiolysis, and amnesia all essential for patient comfort. May be very difficult to mechanically ventilate patients without sedation and analgesia. 2. Agents can be used for other common conditions (lorazepam for acute treatment of seizures and fentanyl for cardiogenic pulmonary edema).
Pulmonary	Bronchodilators	Anticholinergic and β-agonist	1. Minimization of pulmonary secretions. 2. Patients with airway hyperreactivity may be more likely to need critical care. 3. Anticholinergic may have some benefit for nerve agent toxicity as well.
Cardiovascular	Crystalloids	0.9% NaCl or lactated Ringer solution	Relatively inexpensive and first-line therapy for hemodynamic instability and sepsis.
		Hypertonic NaCl (optional)	Less volume required and may have theoretic benefits in sepsis.
	Vasopressor	Institutional preference	No conclusive data supporting efficacy of vasopressors, but relatively inexpensive and severe hypotension despite fluid resuscitation likely to negatively affect patients' outcomes.
Infectious disease	Antimicrobial	Agents consistent with IDSA or ATS guidelines for critically ill community- acquired pneumonia	Most category A agents do not have rapid diagnostic tests, and conditions may be difficult to distinguish from CAP. Patients should be treated for CAP until ruled out with certainty.
Hematologic	Anticoagulant	Institutional preference for thromboembolism prophylaxis in critically ill patients	
Endocrine	Hormone	Insulin	High prevalence of diabetes in population and may be more susceptible to critical illness.

(continued on next page)

Table 1 (continued)			
Organ System	Drug Class	Medication	Reason for Inclusion in Essential Elements of Critical Care
		Hydrocortisone/ fludrocortisones	Benefit in patients with septic shock, but ability to perform and measure cosyntropin stimulation during emergency mass critical care is limited. Debate whether or not benefits patients with septic shock, whose adrenal axis not evaluated.

Abbreviations: ATS, American Thoracic Society; CAP, community-acquired pneumonia; IDSA, Infectious Diseases Society of America.

From Rubinson L, Nuzzo JB, Talmor DS, O'Toole T, Kramer BR, Inglesby TV. Augmentation of hospital critical care capacity after bioterrorist attacks or epidemics: recommendations of the Working Group on Emergency Mass Critical Care. Crit Care Med. 2005 Oct;33(10):2393-403.

for Oxygen use in Adults in Healthcare and Emergency Settings recommends prescribing oxygen to a target saturation of 94% to 98% or 88% to 92% for patient-specific target range for those at risk for hypercapnic respiratory failure.[13] Although adequate supplemental oxygen is fundamental for treatment of hypoxemia but does not treat the underlying cause, there are concerns about the detrimental effects of excessive oxygen or hyperoxia, such as absorption atelectasis, acute lung injury, inflammatory cytokine production, reactive oxygen species, central nervous system toxicity, reduced cardiac output, and cerebral and coronary vasoconstriction.[31] A recent systemic review and meta-analysis of 25 randomized controlled trials found that liberal oxygen therapy (SpO2 >94%–96%) was associated with increased mortality.[32] Inexpensive finger pulse oximeters may be helpful to monitor oxygenation and heart rate when traditional patient monitors are in scarce supply, and thus may be helpful to include in disaster readiness supplies.

SPACE

Initially, patients who require mass critical care will receive care in the ICU. However, with a large number of critically ill patients, it will not take long for the ICU to become full. Hospitals will have to increase their surge capacity by providing critical care in noncritical care spaces. Large academic hospitals tend to have more critical care beds than smaller community hospitals.[33] One approach for hospitals that need additional critical care beds is to use other high-acuity areas of the hospital, such as coronary care units, post anesthesia care units, step-down units, endoscopy and surgical suites, and the emergency room. Ideal rooms for critical care will have supplemental oxygen, telemetry, and room for mechanical ventilation. If the hospital continues to require more critical care rooms, then general wards could be converted to critical care beds. Some advocate transferring noncritical care patients to alternate facilities, such as long-term acute care facilities.[34]

An alternative approach to surge capacity in mass critical care are Acuity Adaptable Units (AAU). In the AAU model, the required level of care is brought to the patient in contrast to the patient transferring to another level of care. This model has primarily been used in the postoperative care of cardiothoracic surgery patients. The patient's room can transform based on the needs of the patient, eliminating the need for patient transfers and reducing medical errors. This AAU model could be used in a disaster where hospital wards are designed to transform from noncritical care beds into critical care beds. In this model, the challenge is having staff that can adapt to the changing medical needs of the patient.[35,36]

One advantage the US military has in mass critical care in the operational settings is the ability to transfer critical care combat patients out of the trauma hospital by critical care air transport to another facility within 24 to 48 hours.[37] In the civilian setting, this can be accomplished by the NDMS but will take some time. A hospital may have very limited ability to divert or transfer in the aftermath of a bioterrorism attack due to the need to prevent further spread of the biological agent.

STRUCTURE

In a mass casualty event, the ICU is one component of the disaster response framework. It is important for hospitals to have staff with critical care experience involved in disaster management. The ICU is a limited resource and the intensivist must have a different mindset in a disaster. There needs to be a paradigm shift away from comprehensive care for everyone to providing the greatest good for the greatest number, predetermined minimal qualifications for survival, predetermined strict ICU admission criteria, and a dynamic protocol based on the event evolution and surge capacity. Unlike most circumstances in which a team of critical care professionals takes care of all patients admitted to the ICU, in a mass casualty incident, there are finite resources of staff and supplies. The intent of triage protocols are to use those finite resources to provide the greatest good for the largest number of patients. This can result in an ethical dilemma for staff when care is not offered to those patients unlikely to recover. Failure to adopt this paradigm shift with respect to triage will result in suboptimal care of the entire cohort of patients and will lead to a deleterious disaster response.[38]

VIRTUAL CRITICAL CARE

Tele-critical care, which is also referred to as virtual critical care, is currently used to fulfill the shortage of critical care providers. Virtual critical care can assist with surge capacity by augmenting critical care staff. Virtual critical care is practiced in a centralized or decentralized model. In the centralized model, the virtual critical care center is at a specific location with 24-hour physician and nursing staff that provide critical care services to many different hospitals. In the decentralized model, virtual critical care consultation is provided by multiple locations to one centralized ICU. Both models can augment critical services in a disaster. Virtual critical care can augment critical care personnel and be organized to provide continuous care, scheduled, or consultative care. An example of scheduled care is nighttime rounding by the virtual intensivist leaving the on-site intensivist to deal with emergent problems. An example of consultative care is the use of a virtual intensivist for management of a specific patient when additional expertise is needed.[39]

The Department of Homeland Security has national planning scenarios that demonstrate the potential role of virtual critical care. The disaster scenarios include a nuclear detonation, anthrax attack, pandemic influenza outbreak, biological attack with the pneumonic plaque, chemical attack with mustard gas, earthquake, bombing, and a hurricane. Virtual critical care can be used in all these scenarios. Examples of the benefits of virtual critical care include remote care reducing the risk of secondary exposure, exposure consultation, triage, ICU monitoring, ARDS management, infectious disease consultation, epidemiology consultation to limit spread, bioterrorism specialist consultation, burn center consultation, radiation sickness specialist consultation, and trauma center consultation.[40]

SUMMARY

The provision of mass critical care requires the ability of a hospital to rapidly increase its patient volume above its normal capacity. The essential 4 components of surge capacity are staff (critical care personnel), stuff (supplies), space (rooms), and structure (management infrastructure). Critical care personnel will have to rely on nonintensivists and civilian caregivers for the provision of critical care services. Staff will have to know the inventory of critical care supplies, what supplies can be reused, and what supply chains are functional in a disaster. Judicious use of scarce supplemental oxygen is essential. Mass critical care requires a different mindset than critical care in day-to-day operations. Finally, virtual critical care/tele-critical care has the potential to augment critical care services in a disaster by supplementing staff but will require secure and reliable telecommunications infrastructure.

ACKNOWLEDGMENTS

The views expressed herein are those of the author(s) and do not necessarily reflect the official policy or position of the Department of the Navy, Department of Defense, or the U.S. Government.

REFERENCES

1. Haupt MT, Bekes CE, Brilli RJ, et al. Guidelines on critical care services and personnel: recommendations based on a system of categorization of three levels of care. Crit Care Med 2003;31(11):2677–83.
2. Nates JL, Nunnally M, Kleinpell R, et al. ICU admission, discharge, and triage guidelines: a framework to enhance clinical operations, development of institutional policies, and further research. Crit Care Med 2016;44(8):1553–602.
3. Weled BJ, Adzhigirey LA, Hodgman TM, et al. Critical care delivery: the importance of process of care and ICU structure to improved outcomes: an update from the American College of Critical Care Medicine Task Force on models of critical care. Crit Care Med 2015;43:1520.
4. Centers for Medicare and Medicaid Services. NHE fact sheet. Available at: https://www.cms.gov/Research-Statistics-Data-and-Systems/Statistics-Trends-and-Reports/NationalHealthExpendData/NHE-Fact-Sheet.html. Accessed May 6, 2016.
5. Vincent GK, Velkoff VA. The next four decades, The older population in the United States: 2010 to 2050. Current Population Reports, P25-1138. Washington, DC: U.S. Census Bureau; 2015. Available at: https://www.census.gov/prod/2010pubs/p25-1138.pdf.
6. Stechmiller JK. The nursing shortage in acute and critical care settings. AACN Clin Issues 2002;13:577–84.
7. Afessa B. Tele-intensive care unit: the horse out of the barn. Crit Care Med 2010; 38(1):292–3.
8. Pronovost PJ, Angus DC, Dorman T, et al. Physician staffing patterns and clinical outcomes in critically ill patients. JAMA 2002;288(17):2151–62.
9. Wilcox M, Chong CA, Niven DJ, et al. Do intensivist staffing patterns influence hospital mortality following ICU admission? A systematic review and meta-analyses. Crit Care Med 2013;41(10):2253–73.

10. Kaji A, Koenig KL, Bey T. Surge capacity for healthcare systems: a conceptual framework. Acad Emerg Med 2006;13:1157–9.

11. Gifford A, Spiro P. Augmenting critical care capacity during a disaster. In: Geiling J, Burns SM, editors. Fundamental disaster management. 3rd edition. Society of Critical Care Medicine; 2008. p. 3-1–3-10.

12. Available at: https://www.jointcommission.org/emergency_management.aspx. Accessed January 19, 2019.

13. Available at: https://www.sccm.org/Fundamentals. Accessed January 19, 2019.

14. Available at: https://www.sccm.org/Fundamentals/FDM. Accessed January 19, 2019.

15. Available at: https://www.facs.org/quality-programs/trauma/education/dmep. Accessed January 19, 2019.

16. Boscarino JA, Adams RE, Figley CR. A prospective cohort study of the effectiveness of employer-sponsored crisis interventions after a major disaster. Int J Emerg Ment Health 2005;7(1):9–22.

17. Available at: https://www.bleedingcontrol.org/. Accessed January 19, 2019.

18. Hick JL, Hanfling D, Burstein JL, et al. Health care facility and community strategies for patient care surge capacity. Ann Emerg Med 2004;44:253–61.

19. Rubinson L, Nuzzo JB, Talmor DS, et al. Augmentation of hospital critical care capacity after bioterrorist attacks or epidemics: recommendations of the Working Group on Emergency Mass Critical Care. Crit Care Med 2005;33(10):2393–403.

20. Davis K, Perry-Moseanko A, Tadlock MD, et al. Successful implementation of low-cost tele-critical care solution by the U.S. Navy: initial experience and recommendations. Mil Med 2017;182(5):e1702–7.

21. Rozovsky F. Emergency credentialing helps disaster response. Hosp Peer Rev 2002;27(5):63–4.

22. Available at: https://www.phe.gov/Preparedness/responders/ndms/ndms-teams/Pages/dmat.aspx. Accessed January 19, 2019.

23. Tosh PK, Feldman H, Christian MD, et al, Task Force for Mass Critical Care. Business and continuity of operations: care of the critically ill and injured during pandemics and disasters: CHEST consensus statement. Chest 2014;146(4 Suppl):e103S–17S.

24. Johannigman JA, Branson RD, Johnson DJ, et al. Out-of-hospital ventilation: bag-valve device vs transport ventilator. Acad Emerg Med 1995;2:719–24.

25. Wilgis J. Strategies for providing mechanical ventilation in a mass casualty incident: distribution versus stockpiling. Respir Care 2008;53(1):96–100.

26. Cardenas-Garcia J, Schaub KF, Belchikov YG, et al. Safety of peripheral intravenous administration of vasoactive medication. J Hosp Med 2015. https://doi.org/10.1002/jhm.2394.

27. Ricard JD, Salomon L, Boyer A, et al. Central or peripheral catheters for initial venous access of ICU patients: a randomized controlled trial. Crit Care Med 2013;41:2108–15.

28. Malatino EM. Strategic national stockpile: overview and ventilator assets. Respir Care 2008;53(1):91–5.

29. Einav S, Hick JL, Hanfling D, et al, Task Force for Mass Critical Care, Task Force for Mass Critical Care. Surge capacity logistics: care of the critically ill and injured during pandemics and disasters: CHEST consensus statement. Chest 2014;146(4 Suppl):e17S–43S.

30. Blakeman TC, Branson RD. Oxygen supplies in disaster management. Respir Care 2013;58(1):173–82.

31. O'Driscoll BR, Howard LS, Earis J, et al, British Thoracic Society Emergency Oxygen Guideline Group, BTS Emergency Oxygen Guideline Development Group. BTS guideline for oxygen use in adults in healthcare and emergency settings. Thorax 2017;72(suppl 1):ii1–90.
32. Chu DK, Kim LH, Young PJ, et al. Mortality and morbidity in acutely ill adults treated with liberal versus conservative oxygen therapy (IOTA): a systematic review and meta-analysis. Lancet 2018;391:1693e705.
33. Wallace DJ, Seymour CW, Kahn JM. Hospital-level changes in adult ICU bed supply in the United States. Crit Care Med 2017;45(1):e67–76.
34. Hick JL, Einav S, Hanfling D, et al. Task force for mass critical care surge capacity principles: care of the critically ill and injured during pandemics and disasters: CHEST consensus statement. Chest 2014;146(4 Suppl):e1S–16S.
35. Hendrich AL, Fay J, Sorrells AK. Effects of acuity-adaptable rooms on flow of patients and delivery of care. Am J Crit Care 2004;13(1):35–45.
36. Chindhy SA, Edwards NM, Rajamanickam V, et al. Acuity adaptable patient care unit system shortens length of stay and improves outcomes in adult cardiac surgery: university of Wisconsin experience. Eur J Cardiothorac Surg 2014;46(1): 49–54.
37. Rice DH, Kotti G, Beninati W. Clinical review: critical care transport and austere critical care. Crit Care 2008;12(2):207.
38. Mahoney EJ, Biffl WL, Cioffi WG. Mass-casualty incidents: how does the ICU prepare? J Intensive Care Med 2008;23(4):219–35.
39. Rolston DM, Meltzer JS. Telemedicine in the intensive care unit: its role in emergencies and disaster management. Crit Care Clin 2015;31:239–55.
40. Jurmain JC, Blancero AJ, Geiling JA, et al. HazBot: development of a telemanipulator robot with haptics for emergency response. Am J Disaster Med 2008; 3(2):87–97.

Triage

Michael D. Christian, MD, MSc, FRCPC

KEYWORDS

- Triage • Mass casualty incident • Crisis response

KEY POINTS

- Triage decision making is critical for a successful response to a mass casualty incident.
- How triage is applied differs across the surge response spectrum from conventional to crisis response.
- Disaster triage is a complex topic with which most clinicians have limited experience and often have difficulty in making the shift from the patient to population perspective to understand it well.

WHAT IS TRIAGE?

Intensive care clinicians are often uncertain as to what triage truly means and entails in a disaster situation. Their uncertainty likely stems from a lack of experience among clinicians in conducting triage in this context[1] combined with a tendency to confuse it with the concepts of "triage" applied on a routine basis within the emergency room (ER)[2] of hospitals or access to specialist services, such as cardiac catheterization and stroke services.

To understand the meaning of triage in a disaster setting, it is helpful to consider the origins of the word. Originating from the French verb "trier" meaning "to sort," it was first used in the fifteenth century marketplaces in England and France to refer to grouping goods by quality and price.[1–5] Implicit in this early application of the term is the second component of triage, which is to assign some ranked value or priority to what is being sorted (**Fig. 1**). This prioritization aspect of triage is what is practiced on a routine basis in the ER and elsewhere but distinctly different from the full extent of triage used in a disaster.[6] In disasters, in addition to sorting and prioritizing patients, triage also includes allocating scarce resources in order to "do the greatest good for the greatest number" (**Box 1**).[1,2,4–10] Although this phrase easily slips off the tongue, many overlook its profound implications implicit in shifting decision making from a focus on individual patient outcomes to population-level outcomes.[4,5,7] Although many clinicians have day-to-day experience with prioritizing patients for the benefit of that individual patient, very few clinicians have experience with population-level decision making during periods of resource scarcity.[1,6]

London's Air Ambulance, Bart's Health NHS Trust, Helipad, Royal London Hospital, Whitechapel Road, Whitechapel, London E1 1BB, UK
E-mail address: michael.christian@utoronto.ca

Crit Care Clin 35 (2019) 575–589
https://doi.org/10.1016/j.ccc.2019.06.009   criticalcare.theclinics.com

Priority Group			Description
Number	Name	Color	
P1	Emergency/Immediate	Red	Patients who have life-threatening injuries that are treatable with a minimum amount of time, personnel, and supplies. These patients also have a good chance of recovery.
P2	Urgent	Yellow	Indicates that treatment may be delayed for a limited period of time without significant mortality or in the ICU setting patients for whom life support may or may not change their outcome given the severity of their illness.
P3	Delayed	Green	Patients with minor injuries whose treatment may be delayed until the patients in the other categories have been dealt with or patients who do not require ICU admission for the provision of life support.
P4	Expectant	Blue	Patients who have injuries requiring extensive treatment that exceeds the medical resources available in the situation or for whom life support is considered futile.
--	Dead	Black	Patients who are in cardiac arrest and for which resuscitation efforts are not going to be provided.

Fig. 1. Priority groups commonly used in triage for health care. (*Data from* Refs.[1,2,51,84])

Bridging the concept between patients and populations outcomes are the terms "undertriage" and "overtriage."[2,11–15] In undertriage. a patient is not recognized to be as sick or injured as they truly are, resulting in delayed treatment impacting the chance of survival for the individual as well as the overall survival rate within the population. With overtriage, a patient is misidentified as being more ill or injured than they actually are, and their care is prioritized higher than others who are actually in greater need. As a result of both the delayed treatment to the individual patients lower in the queue and the potentially inappropriate consumption of limited resources (staff, stuff, or space), the overall population outcome is worse.

When making triage decisions in resource-scarce situations, it is important to keep a few key concepts in mind. When evaluating a potential benefit of a treatment to a patient, one is attempting to determine the incremental benefit[7,15,16] of that treatment compared with receiving a less resource-intensive or delayed treatment, but rarely does this ever mean no treatment. For example, it cannot be simply assumed that if a patient does not receive admission to intensive care and the provision of life support that they will certainly die.[17] Furthermore, what is being considered is not a binary outcome between death and survival but rather the probability of death across an entire range of treatment options.[7] Finally, it is important to remember that for both patients and society, survival in of itself is not the only outcome of concern; equally important is the quality of life for those who survive. Thus, the key factors being considered when making disaster triage decisions need to include survival, quality of life, and the resources necessary to achieve these outcomes (**Box 2**).[18]

Box 1
Components of disaster triage

Sorting

Prioritizing

Allocating resources

Box 2
Disaster triage outcome considerations
Survival
Quality of life
Resource consumption
Data from Christian MD, Fowler R, Muller MP, et al. Critical care resource allocation: trying to PREEDICCT outcomes without a crystal ball. Critical Care. 2013;17(1):3.

WHEN TO TRIAGE

The Task Force for Mass Critical Care recommends that "in the event of an incident with mass critical care casualties, all hospitals within a defined geographic/administrative region, health authority, or health-care coalition implement a uniform triage process should critical care resources become scarce."[16] A subtler and more important nuance to this question is when to move from routine triage to disaster triage. The decision to implement "disaster triage" involves the additional component of resource allocation implicit in the meaning of the term "disaster." A disaster can be defined as an event that results in injuries or loss of life and results in a demand for services that exceeds available resources.[19] However, in terms of the health care response to an event, this binary concept of either being in a disaster or not is less helpful and likely impairs the response; thus, it is much more useful and common to consider the concepts of surge management.[20–23] Applying these principles, the clinician scales response strategies (conventional, contingency, or crisis) to the magnitude of the surge based on the balance between resource demand and supply, which is context dependent and will vary from incident to incident. In situations of minor or moderate surge whereby conventional and contingency strategies are used, the standard of care for patients remains relatively comparable to normal,[24] and thus, only routine triage (sorting and prioritizing) should occur (**Fig. 2**). It is only during a major surge,

Magnitude of Surge		Minor	Moderate	Major (overwhelming)
Standard of care		Conventional	Contingency	Crisis
Response Strategies		Conserve Substitute	Conserve Substitute Adapt Re-use	Conserve Substitute Adapt Re-use Reallocate
Type of triage		Routine	Routine	Disaster
Components of triage in use	Sort	★	★	★
	Prioritize	★	★	★
	Resource Allocation	--	--	★

Fig. 2. Application of triage based on magnitude of surge. (*Adapted from* Christian, M. D., et al. (2014). Introduction and executive summary: care of the critically ill and injured during pandemics and disasters: CHEST consensus statement. Chest 146(4 Suppl): 8S-34S; and *Data from* Hick JL, Barbera JA, Kelen GD. Refining surge capacity: conventional, contingency, and crisis capacity. Disaster Med Public Health Prep. 2009;3(5_suppl):S59-S67.)

when resources are, or will be, overwhelmed do crisis standards of care[25] and response strategies involving the allocation (rationing) of resources come into play, necessitating "disaster triage."[16]

Making the transition to disaster triage, shifting the focus to population outcomes and implementing resource allocation processes, is a decision that carries with it significant implications for all involved (patients, clinicians, hospitals, and society) and thus requires appropriate approvals and governance.[15] In most well-resourced societies, patients have access to health care resources even in situations wherein there are vanishingly small chances of them benefiting. Once a decision is made to implement disaster triage, many of these patients will have their access to these resources restricted with potential consequences for them.[2] In addition, this transition is very difficult for clinicians who likely have never faced such situations in their careers.[1,26] Patients who are not triaged to immediate treatment should be reevaluated regularly and retriaged if their condition changes or the resource situation improves. All patients should receive some form of treatment, at a minimum, palliative care.[1,2,27]

DIFFERENT TYPES OF DISASTER TRIAGE

The most common classification of triage is based on the location and level of care at which the triage takes place. Primary, secondary, and tertiary triage (**Table 1**) can be conducted for critically ill and injured patients and is the focus of this article. Other forms of triage critical care clinicians should also be aware of include public health triage and reverse triage.[1,16,28,29] Public health triage refers to triage protocols that distribute vaccinations or countermeasures in the event of an outbreak, pandemic, terrorism incident or biowarfare.[9,30–33] Effective public health triage may decreased demand on critical care resources. Reverse triage[34–36] is used to discharge patients at low risk of adverse events from either the intensive care unit (ICU) or hospital wards in turn to create ICU capacity.

Regardless of the type of disaster, triage must address all sources of demand for critical care, not only those demands associated with the surge event itself.[37] For example, following a natural disaster or terrorism attack creating an influx of trauma patients, the triage system must also be able to fairly allocate critical care resources to patients with medical conditions unrelated to the incident, such as respiratory failure from acute respiratory distress syndrome owing to sepsis or a woman with postpartum hemorrhage.[2,38]

Primary Triage

Primary triage occurs in the field with the aim of determining priorities for treatment on scene and transport of patients to hospital. Although a large number of adult and

Table 1 Classification of triage by location		
Triage Type	Location	Priorities Addressed
Primary	Field	Who to immediately treat on scene (triage sieve) and priorities for evacuation from scene (triage sort)
Secondary	Entry to ER	Who to prioritize for resuscitation and disposition to treatment areas within the ER and/or admission to hospital ward
Tertiary	Exit from ER or entry to ICU/OR	Who to prioritize for definitive/critical care (OR and admission to ICU)

pediatric protocols[2,38–40] have been developed, best practice in primary triage remains controversial because no protocol has been prospectively validated in a disaster[39,41] or accepted as being superior to all others.[37,40] Primary triage of the critically injured patient may be one of the most important decision points impacting the outcome for critically ill and injured patients.[2] With the advances of Major Trauma Systems and wide spread utilization of Trauma Triage Tools on a routine basis, there have been recent suggestions made to restrict primary triage during conventional and contingency responses to a binary decision (triage to major trauma center vs triage to a regular ER).[42] Two priority triage however is not a new concept, some military investigators have been advocating simplification of field triage for many years.[1] Although Critical Care Physicians have often not been involved in primary triage in the past, with the general recognition of the need for critical care to occur outside of the walls of the ICU wherever patients need it, this is an area Critical Care Physicians should become more engaged in planning, overseeing, and delivering.

Secondary Triage

The objective of secondary triage varies depending on the nature of the incident. In a sudden onset[43] kinetic event, such as an earthquake, bombing, or transport incident, where trauma is the primary "disease" being managed, the key objective of secondary triage is to determine the priority for treating patients arriving at the emergency department (ED). In the event of a delayed onset event, such as a pandemic or public health emergency, wherein the time course of the disease being treated is also more protracted, the primary objective of secondary triage is to determine who to admit to hospital because they are at high risk of deteriorating and may require intensive care or other high-dependency resources. In either case, one can think of secondary triage as occurring at the "front door" of the hospital.

Very few protocols have been developed to support secondary triage. Some hospitals apply primary triage protocols, such as simple triage and rapid treatment (START), for secondary triage; however, understandably, they perform poorly in this setting.[44] Duplicating primary triage in hospital is not only unlikely to be effective for achieving the different objectives of secondary triage but also highly inefficient and fails to take into account the additional information available on which to base a secondary triage decision. In most situations, secondary triage is conducted by a single senior physician or surgeon or group of senior physicians or surgeons drawn from a variety of backgrounds, including emergency medicine, intensive care, or trauma surgery.[28,45–47] Toida and colleagues[44] developed the Pediatric Physiological and Anatomical Triage Score specifically for pediatric secondary triage for trauma and CBRNE (chemical, biological, radiological, nuclear, and explosive) -related disasters. Pneumonia severity scores[48,49] have been investigated for secondary triage in pandemics but found to perform poorly. However, secondary triage criteria established by the UK health department specifically for a pandemic performed well in studies.[48]

Tertiary Triage

Tertiary triage occurs within the hospital with the objective of prioritizing patients, and if required allocating resources, for definitive care (operations or interventional radiology procedures) and intensive care (life support therapies). Tertiary triage decisions are generally more complex than earlier triage decisions given the larger amount of information available from multiple assessment points and investigations. Trauma tertiary triage is typically conducted by a senior clinician, usually a surgeon, anesthetist, or intensivist, based on their clinical experience.[28,36] Following the outbreak of severe acute respiratory syndrome[50] in 2003 and the development of the first protocol[51] for

ICU tertiary triage, there has been a significant amount of work to further develop such protocols.[16,18,29,52–61]

Most well-developed and evaluated ICU triage protocols[16,29,51,57,58,60,61] have used inclusion and exclusion criteria in combination with the sequential organ failure score (SOFA). In a conventional or contingency situation, when there is not an absolute short-fall of resources, the inclusion criteria for admission to ICU in most units will be patients who are at high risk of deteriorating and requiring initiation of life support or who are already receiving life support. When a shift is made to a crisis response, the inclusion criteria threshold changes to those who have already declared themselves to abso-lutely require life support. Similarly, exclusion criteria, which exist even during conven-tional and contingency situations,[15,62,63] shift during a crisis such that patients with either baseline conditions or severity of illness/injury that places them in the realm of futility for immediate to short-term survival may be excluded. The use of the SOFA score in these protocols is not without controversy.[64–67] However, the latest iterations of an ICU triage protocol[57] developed by the Influenza Pandemic ICU Triage Study In-vestigators of the Australian and New Zealand Intensive Care Society clinical trials group improve on prior attempts and show significant promise.

To date, there are no reported incidents wherein any of these ICU triage protocols have been actively implemented to allocate scarce resources. However, when Hurri-cane Sandy struck New York City, Dr Laura Evans reported[68] that the Ontario ICU Triage Protocol provided an important framework to plan if allocation was required for electrical power for ventilators. During the H1N1 pandemic, governments in Canada, the United Kingdom, and New Zealand established triage protocols, based on the Ontario protocol,[51] to be implemented if ICU resources were overwhelmed.[58,66]

HOW TO TRIAGE AND WHO SHOULD DO IT

There are several key considerations when planning and delivering triage. These con-siderations include the critical decisions of who to select to do triage, whether triage should be conducted by individuals or teams, whether they should follow protocols or act on their clinical intuition, and finally, if using protocols, on what should the proto-cols be based.

Who Should Conduct Triage?

Effective triage depends on careful choice as to who should make triage decisions.[2] As with all aspects of managing a major incident, compromises may have to be made based on the resources available and the context of the situation. Consistently, experts (and the public[69]) recommend that triage in mass casualty situations should be conducted by highly experienced physicians, who possess the necessary skill set (**Box 3**).[1,2,16,28,29,45–47,51,53,54,61,70–73] Having experienced physicians conduct triage applies to triage at all levels, including primary triage in the field. Previously, it was thought that in well-developed Emergency Medical Systems paramedics alone could undertake primary triage, and there was a limited role for physicians in this setting.[2] However, more recent experience[28,74] and data show the benefit of properly trained and equipped prehospital physicians in primary triage, in particular when there are delays in evacuating patients from the scene to hospital.[46] When an experienced physician/surgeon is not available to triage, then the next most clinically trained and experienced providers should undertake triage.

There are several reasons senior physicians and surgeons are recommended (and found to perform better[6,75]) over other less highly trained or experienced providers. First, there is some evidence that their knowledge and understanding of triage may

Box 3
Essential triage officer skills
Extensive clinical experience
Strong leadership
Effective communication
Agile decision making

be better,[6] but that seems to be a minor component. Likely the critical factor is their clinical experience impacting their ability to rapidly identify "sick from well," combined with their ability to understand patients' overall clinical course and treatment needs (the "big picture").[1] Providers such as paramedics rarely are afforded the opportunity to have longer-term follow-up on their patients or to see how they progress over the course of their acute illness/injury or respond to definitive treatments. Just as it is important for the surgeon or intensivist doing tertiary triage to understand what will happen in the operating room (OR)/ICU, so too will triage be most effective if primary triage decisions are informed by an understanding of what resources the patient requires on arrival to hospital and the systems in place to provide them. Finally, senior physicians, in particular, intensivists and emergency medicine physicians who manage multiple patients in large ICUs or EDs on a daily basis, are well accustomed and experienced in making complex, critical decisions with limited information.[76–79] This type of experience makes them uniquely well suited for both triage and leadership in major incidents.

Given that the key objective of the triage officer is to save the most lives, the senior triage officer should have ultimate control over all resources within their area of operation (department) and thus ultimately command the situation. Even in the military, Swan and Swan[1] point out that "In time of triage, the triage officer outranks the hospital commander, in practice, and this needs to be clearly understood by all involved, including the commanding officer!"[1] At the organizational level, it is also important to ensure a similarly experienced physician or surgeon is in command to appropriately support the department-level triage officers.[45]

Should Individuals or Teams Triage?

Although it seems straightforward, this question is not as simple as it sounds. The crux of the issue is whether triage decisions, at the coal face in the midst of a mass casualty situation, should be made by an individual or a committee. Most recommendations suggest an individual triage officer[1,2,16,28,29,45–47,51,53,70–73] rather than a committee.[54,60] However, even in those studies that do recommend a single person ultimately makes the triage decision, most recommend that a multidisciplinary team work in conjunction with and support the triage officer through obtaining information, undertaking assessments, and so forth. Following good leadership principles, the triage officer should take input from his/her team members; thus, having a single final decision maker does not mean decisions are made in isolation. Multiple triage officers (and supporting teams) may be required to manage casualty volumes. Although some advocate committee-based triage decisions, it is unlikely that primary, secondary, or tertiary triage decisions could ever be effectively implemented on scale with the required time dependencies for such decisions, including decisions regarding critical care in a mass casualty incident. Reverse triage decisions, including the withdrawal of life support, may be more amenable to a committee-type decision given the lack of time pressures for these decisions.

Should Protocols Be Used for Triage?

The primary benefits of using a protocol for triage are 2-fold: first, it provides a decision support aid in a time of crisis to improve performance; second, if designed and applied appropriately, it should improve consistency of decisions made as well as improve outcomes. For any triage protocol to be successful, it must be able to distinguish those most in need and most likely to benefit from therapy. Poorly performing protocols may lead to worse outcomes than other options, such as first come, first served.[80] The alternative to using a protocol is to rely solely on clinician intuition, "gut instinct," for triage decisions.[2,40,70]

Much work has recently been undertaken attempting to develop protocols to support tertiary triage. Given that any ICU triage protocol must apply to all patients being considered for ICU admission, most of the protocols have been based on physiologic prognostic scores, such as the SOFA score.[16,29,51,57,58,60,81] Although this addresses the need for a score that applies to all, there is concern about certain subjective aspects of the SOFA score (including Glasgow Coma Scale measurement and level of inotrope support), its lack of applicability for pediatric patients,[82] as well as concerns about the performance of the score.[65,67,83] However, the studies questioning SOFA performance have done so based on individual patient outcome analyses not population-level outcomes (overall survival), which should be the basis of triage evaluations.[7] It may be possible to combine multiple disease-specific scores, such as the injury severity score (ISS), revised trauma score (RTS), burn scores, or pneumonia scores, for triage using a computer decision support algorithm and common outcome measures.[18] However, current evidence suggests the RTS[72] and ISS[84] perform poorly for triage.

WHAT ARE THE ETHICS OF TRIAGE AND HOW TO GOVERN TRIAGE?

A review of the ethics of triage is a complete article unto itself, and several excellent reviews already exist.[85–88] Key concepts related to the ethics of triage are listed in **Table 2**. Although there is no single agreed upon "right" ethical principle on which

Table 2
Ethical guide for pandemic planning

Substantive Values to Guide Ethical Decision Making[1]	Procedural Values to Guide Ethical Decision Making[1]	Ethical Principles Possible to Inform Triage
• Individual liberty • Protection of the public from harm • Proportionality • Privacy • Duty to provide care • Reciprocity • Equity • Trust • Solidarity • Stewardship	• Reasonableness • Transparency • Inclusiveness • Responsiveness • Accountability	• Utilitarian: "greatest good for the greatest number" • Egalitarian: "allocation based on need" • Libertarian: "protection of individual liberty & patient choice" social benefit • Communitarian: "respect for social & cultural values" • Life cycle: "fair innings or years of life saved"

Data from University of Toronto Joint Centre for Bioethics Pandemic Influenza Working Group. *Stand on Guard for Thee. Ethical considerations in preparedness planning for pandemic influenza.* Toronto: University of Toronto;2005 to base triage,[54] it is generally accepted that population (public health) ethical frameworks should be used rather than the traditional framework of medical ethics. Many clinicians can find this conceptual transition difficult to make. Further complicating matters is that ethical perspectives vary at the societal level around the world on many topics, including their views on the role of clinicians in decision making and use of "lotteries" rather than triage for the allocation of scarce resources.[26,60,69,89]

Effective governance of triage requires a legal basis authorizing its application as well as infrastructure mechanisms to ensure it is conducted appropriately (**Box 4**). Several publications by public health legal experts explore in detail the issues surrounding the legislative framework and other legal issues related to disaster triage.[90–92] Unfortunately, the legal and governance aspects of triage are often neglected by governments, and health care workers will be left to manage in a disaster with limited support and a lack of guidance. Addressing the gaps in these areas should be a priority for government officials and emergency planners.

WHAT RESEARCH IS REQUIRED ON TRIAGE?

The research literature on triage in disasters remains relatively limited, and what data are available are thought to be of low quality.[37,93] Some notable exceptions are recent examples of high-quality research into ICU triage ethics[26,69] and triage protocol development.[57,58] To date, there has been no prospective validation of the major incident triage tools during a major incident.[39] There are two common errors found among the triage research literature worth highlighting with the hope to prevent others from making similar mistakes in the future. The first error is to attempt to use general ICU populations from non-resource-scarce scenarios to test or derive triage protocols for use in mass casualty situations and the second is to fail to understand the different aims of secondary and tertiary triage.

The research by Morton and colleagues[94] provide an example of both errors in that they attempt to evaluate the Ontario Triage Protocol[51] using a population that includes patients who are not admitted to intensive care as well as those in ICU but who do not require life support. Thus, they include a population that does not meet the inclusion criteria for which the Ontario Triage Protocol was designed. In addition, the focus of Morton's research question is to "predict the need for mechanical ventilation and

---

Box 4
Infrastructure and processes required for effective triage governance

- Legislative framework for the allocation of scarce resources in a disaster

- Uniform triage policies and processes across a geographic or administrative region

- Mechanism for a public body with adequate situational awareness and legal authority to initiate rationing (resource allocation) aspect of triage when resources have become scarce

- System to develop triage policies/protocols and provide oversight of triage decisions

- Effective command and control process (eg, Incident Management System)

- Effective communication system and process for sharing situational awareness of resource status

- Training for triage officers

- Psychological support system for triage officers and health care workers

Data from Christian MD, Sprung CL, King MA, et al. Triage: Care of the Critically Ill and Injured During Pandemics and Disasters: CHEST Consensus Statement. *Chest.* 2014;146(4 Suppl):e61S-74S.

critical care admission." As discussed earlier, this is posed as an erroneous question of tertiary triage in a mass casualty situation and would actually guide who to prioritize for hospital admission (secondary triage). Rather, tertiary triage occurs among those who have already declared themselves to require life support and aims to predict who will benefit from it most and lead to the overall highest survival in the population. The work by Adeniji and Cusack[95] provides another example of these same errors being made.[95] The first step to conducting high-quality research in triage is to understand the underlying principles of triage.

SUMMARY

Triage decision making is critical for a successful response to a mass casualty incident. How triage is applied differs across the surge response spectrum from conventional to crisis response. Mass casualty triage is a complex topic with which most clinicians have limited experience and with which most clinicians often have difficulty in making the shift from the patient to population perspective to understand it well. Further training and research are necessary to advance this field and better prepare intensive care clinicians to respond to disasters.

REFERENCES

1. Swan KG, Swan KG Jr. Triage: the past revisited. Mil Med 1996;161(8):448–52.
2. Kennedy K, Aghababian RV, Gans L, et al. Triage: techniques and applications in decision making. Ann Emerg Med 1996;28(2):136–44.
3. Nakao H, Ukai I, Kotani J. A review of the history of the origin of triage from a disaster medicine perspective. Acute Med Surg 2017;4(4):379–84.
4. Iserson KV, Moskop JC. Triage in medicine, part I: concept, history, and types. Ann Emerg Med 2007;49(3):275–81.
5. Veatch RM. Disaster preparedness and triage: justice and the common good. Mt Sinai J Med 2005;72(4):236–41.
6. Janousek JT, Jackson DE, De Lorenzo RA, et al. Mass casualty triage knowledge of military medical personnel. Mil Med 1999;164(5):332–5.
7. Gomersall CD, Joynt GM. What is the benefit in triage? Crit Care Med 2011;39(4): 911–2.
8. Baker MS. Creating order from chaos: part I: triage, initial care, and tactical considerations in mass casualty and disaster response. Mil Med 2007;172(3):232–6.
9. Burkle FM. Population-based triage management in response to surge-capacity requirements during a large-scale bioevent disaster. Acad Emerg Med 2006; 13(11):1118–29.
10. Moskop JC, Iserson KV. Triage in medicine, part II: underlying values and principles. Ann Emerg Med 2007;49(3):282–7.
11. Armstrong JH, Hammond J, Hirshberg A, et al. Is overtriage associated with increased mortality? The evidence says "yes". Disaster Med Public Health Prep 2008;2(1):4–5 [author reply: 5–6].
12. Hupert N, Hollingsworth E, Xiong W. Is overtriage associated with increased mortality? Insights from a simulation model of mass casualty trauma care. Disaster Med Public Health Prep 2007;1(1 Suppl):S14–24.
13. Frykberg ER. Medical management of disasters and mass casualties from terrorist bombings: how can we cope? J Trauma 2002;53(2):201–12.
14. Frykberg ER. Terrorist bombings in Madrid. Crit Care 2005;9(1):20–2.

15. Blanch L, Abillama FF, Amin P, et al. Triage decisions for ICU admission: report from the Task Force of the World Federation of Societies of Intensive and Critical Care Medicine. J Crit Care 2016;36:301–5.
16. Christian MD, Sprung CL, King MA, et al. Triage: care of the critically ill and injured during pandemics and disasters: CHEST consensus statement. Chest 2014;146(4 Suppl):e61S–74S.
17. Joynt GM, Gomersall CD, Tan P, et al. Prospective evaluation of patients refused admission to an intensive care unit: triage, futility and outcome. Intensive Care Med 2001;27(9):1459–65.
18. Christian MD, Fowler R, Muller MP, et al. Critical care resource allocation: trying to PREEDICCT outcomes without a crystal ball. Crit Care 2013;17(1):3.
19. Lewis CP, Aghababian RV. Disaster planning, Part I. Overview of hospital and emergency department planning for internal and external disasters. Emerg Med Clin North Am 1996;14(2):439–52.
20. Hick JL, Barbera JA, Kelen GD. Refining surge capacity: conventional, contingency, and crisis capacity. Disaster Med Public Health Prep 2009;3(2 Suppl):S59–67.
21. Hick JL, Christian MD, Sprung CL. Chapter 2. Surge capacity and infrastructure considerations for mass critical care. Recommendations and standard operating procedures for intensive care unit and hospital preparations for an influenza epidemic or mass disaster. Intensive Care Med 2010;36(Suppl 1):S11–20.
22. Hick JL, Einav S, Hanfling D, et al. Surge capacity principles: care of the critically ill and injured during pandemics and disasters: CHEST consensus statement. Chest 2014;146(4 Suppl):e1S–16S.
23. Hick JL, Hanfling D, Burstein JL, et al. Health care facility and community strategies for patient care surge capacity. Ann Emerg Med 2004;44(3):253–61.
24. Christian MD, Devereaux AV, Dichter JR, et al. Introduction and executive summary: care of the critically ill and injured during pandemics and disasters: CHEST consensus statement. Chest 2014;146(4 Suppl):8S–34S.
25. Altevogt BM, Institute of Medicine (U.S.), Committee on Guidance for Establishing Standards of Care for Use in Disaster Situations. Guidance for establishing crisis standards of care for use in disaster situations: a letter report. Washington, DC: National Academies Press; 2009.
26. Biddison ELD, Gwon HS, Schoch-Spana M, et al. Scarce resource allocation during disasters: a mixed-method community engagement study. Chest 2018;153(1):187–95.
27. Nouvet E, Sivaram M, Bezanson K, et al. Palliative care in humanitarian crises: a review of the literature. Int J Humanitarian Action 2018;3(1):5.
28. Orban JC, Quintard H, Ichai C. ICU specialists facing terrorist attack: the Nice experience. Intensive Care Med 2017;43(5):683–5.
29. Devereaux AV, Dichter JR, Christian MD, et al. Definitive care for the critically ill during a disaster: a framework for allocation of scarce resources in mass critical care: from a Task Force for Mass Critical Care summit meeting, January 26-27, 2007, Chicago, IL. Chest 2008;133(5 Suppl):51S–66S.
30. Howard MJ, Brillman JC, Burkle FM. Infectious disease emergencies in disasters. Emerg Med Clin North Am 1996;14(2):413–28.
31. Klein KR, Pepe PE, Burkle FM, et al. Evolving need for alternative triage management in public health emergencies: a Hurricane Katrina case study. Disaster Med Public Health Prep 2008;2(Suppl 1):S40–4.

32. Sox HC. A triage algorithm for inhalational anthrax. Ann Intern Med 2003; 139(5 Pt 1):379–81.
33. Cone DC, Koenig KL. Mass casualty triage in the chemical, biological, radiological, or nuclear environment. Eur J Emerg Med 2005;12(6):287–302.
34. Satterthwaite PS, Atkinson CJ. Using 'reverse triage' to create hospital surge capacity: Royal Darwin Hospital's response to the Ashmore Reef disaster. Emerg Med J 2012;29(2):160–2.
35. Kelen GD, Troncoso R, Trebach J, et al. Effect of reverse triage on creation of surge capacity in a pediatric hospital. JAMA Pediatr 2017;171(4):e164829.
36. Einav S, Hick JL, Hanfling D, et al. Surge capacity logistics: care of the critically ill and injured during pandemics and disasters: CHEST consensus statement. Chest 2014;146(4 Suppl):e17S–43S.
37. Timbie JW, Ringel JS, Fox DS, et al. Systematic review of strategies to manage and allocate scarce resources during mass casualty events. Ann Emerg Med 2013;61(6):677–89.e101.
38. Arshad FH, Williams A, Asaeda G, et al. A modified simple triage and rapid treatment algorithm from the New York City (USA) Fire Department. Prehosp Disaster Med 2015;30(2):199–204.
39. Vassallo J, Beavis J, Smith JE, et al. Major incident triage: derivation and comparative analysis of the modified physiological triage tool (MPTT). Injury 2017;48(5): 992–9.
40. Klein KR, Burkle FM Jr, Swienton R, et al. Qualitative analysis of surveyed emergency responders and the identified factors that affect first stage of primary triage decision-making of mass casualty incidents. PLoS Curr 2016;8 [pii:ecurrents.dis.d69dafcfb3ad8be88b3e655bd38fba84].
41. Jenkins JL, McCarthy ML, Sauer LM, et al. Mass-casualty triage: time for an evidence-based approach. Prehosp Disaster Med 2008;23(1):3–8.
42. Pan London Major Trauma Networks: response to mass casualty incident. London: Center for Trauma Sciences; 2016.
43. Devereaux A, Christian MD, Dichter JR, et al, Care TFfMC. Summary of suggestions from the task force for mass critical care summit, January 26-27, 2007. Chest 2008;133(5 Suppl):1S–7S.
44. Toida C, Muguruma T, Abe T, et al. Introduction of pediatric physiological and anatomical triage score in mass-casualty incident. Prehosp Disaster Med 2018; 33(2):147–52.
45. Einav S, Spira RM, Hersch M, et al. Surgeon and hospital leadership during terrorist-related multiple-casualty events: a coup d'etat. Arch Surg 2006;141(8): 815–22.
46. Hick JL, Hanfling D, Cantrill SV. Allocating scarce resources in disasters: emergency department principles. Ann Emerg Med 2012;59(3):177–87.
47. Shirley PJ, Mandersloot G. Clinical review: the role of the intensive care physician in mass casualty incidents: planning, organisation, and leadership. Crit Care 2008;12(3):214.
48. Myles PR, Semple MG, Lim WS, et al. Predictors of clinical outcome in a national hospitalised cohort across both waves of the influenza A/H1N1 pandemic 2009-2010 in the UK. Thorax 2012;67(8):709–17.
49. Commons RJ, Denholm J. Triaging pandemic flu: pneumonia severity scores are not the answer. Int J Tuberc Lung Dis 2012;16(5):670–3.
50. Christian MD, Poutanen SM, Loutfy MR, et al. Severe acute respiratory syndrome. Clin Infect Dis 2004;38(10):1420–7.

51. Christian MD, Hawryluck L, Wax RS, et al. Development of a triage protocol for critical care during an influenza pandemic. CMAJ 2006;175(11):1377–81.
52. Christian MD, Hamielec C, Lazar NM, et al. A retrospective cohort pilot study to evaluate a triage tool for use in a pandemic. Crit Care 2009;13(5):R170.
53. Christian MD, Toltzis P, Kanter RK, et al. Treatment and triage recommendations for pediatric emergency mass critical care. Pediatr Crit Care Med 2011;12(6): S109–19.
54. Eastman N, Philips B, Rhodes A. Triaging for adult critical care in the event of overwhelming need. Intensive Care Med 2010;36(6):1076–82.
55. Powell T, Christ KC, Birkhead GS. Allocation of ventilators in a public health disaster. Disaster Med Public Health Prep 2008;2(1):20–6.
56. Rubinson L, Christian MD. Allocating mechanical ventilators during mass respiratory failure: kudos to New York State, but more work to be done. Disaster Med Public Health Prep 2008;2(1):7–10.
57. Cheung W, Myburgh J, Seppelt IM, et al. Development and evaluation of an influenza pandemic intensive care unit triage protocol. Crit Care Resusc 2012;14(3): 185–90.
58. Cheung WK, Myburgh J, Seppelt IM, et al. A multicentre evaluation of two intensive care unit triage protocols for use in an influenza pandemic. Med J Aust 2012; 197(3):178–81.
59. Gall C, Wetzel R, Kolker A, et al. Pediatric triage in a severe pandemic: maximizing survival by establishing triage thresholds. Crit Care Med 2016;44(9): 1762–8.
60. Daugherty Biddison EL, Faden R, Gwon HS, et al. Too many patients...a framework to guide statewide allocation of scarce mechanical ventilation during disasters. Chest 2018;155(4):848–54.
61. Christian MD, Joynt GM, Hick JL, et al. Chapter 7. Critical care triage. Recommendations and standard operating procedures for intensive care unit and hospital preparations for an influenza epidemic or mass disaster. Intensive Care Med 2010;36(Suppl 1):S55–64.
62. Zawacki BE. ICU physician's ethical role in distributing scarce resources. Crit Care Med 1985;13(1):57–60.
63. Fair allocation of intensive care unit resources. American Thoracic Society. Am J Respir Crit Care Med 1997;156(4 Pt 1):1282–301.
64. Zygun DA, Laupland KB, Fick GH, et al. Limited ability of SOFA and MOD scores to discriminate outcome: a prospective evaluation in 1,436 patients. Can J Anaesth 2005;52(3):302–8.
65. Khan Z, Hulme J, Sherwood N. An assessment of the validity of SOFA score based triage in H1N1 critically ill patients during an influenza pandemic. Anaesthesia 2009;64(12):1283–8.
66. Guest T, Tantam G, Donlin N, et al. An observational cohort study of triage for critical care provision during pandemic influenza: 'clipboard physicians' or 'evidenced based medicine'? Anaesthesia 2009;64(11):1199–206.
67. Shahpori R, Stelfox HT, Doig CJ, et al. Sequential organ failure assessment in H1N1 pandemic planning. Crit Care Med 2011;39(4):827–32.
68. McKnight W. Ready or not? Most ICUs not as prepared for disaster as they think. Chest Physician. November 25, 2013.
69. Cheung W, Myburgh J, McGuinness S, et al. A cross-sectional survey of Australian and New Zealand public opinion on methods to triage intensive care patients in an influenza pandemic. Crit Care Resusc 2017;19(3):254–65.

70. Hashimoto A, Ueda T, Kuboyama K, et al. Application of a first impression triage in the Japan railway west disaster. Acta Med Okayama 2013;67(3):171–6.

71. Shirley PJ. Critical care delivery: the experience of a civilian terrorist attack. J R Army Med Corps 2006;152(1):17–21.

72. Burkle FM Jr, Newland C, Orebaugh S, et al. Emergency medicine in the Persian Gulf War—part 2. Triage methodology and lessons learned. Ann Emerg Med 1994;23(4):748–54.

73. Burkle FM Jr, Orebaugh S, Barendse BR. Emergency medicine in the Persian Gulf War–part 1: preparations for triage and combat casualty care. Ann Emerg Med 1994;23(4):742–7.

74. Blank-Reid C, Santora TA. Developing and implementing a surgical response and physician triage team. Disaster Manag Response 2003;1(2):41–5.

75. Follmann A, Ohligs M, Hochhausen N, et al. Technical support by smart glasses during a mass casualty incident: a randomized controlled simulation trial on technically assisted triage and telemedical app use in disaster medicine. J Med Internet Res 2019;21(1):e11939.

76. Reader TW, Flin R, Cuthbertson BH. Team leadership in the intensive care unit: the perspective of specialists. Crit Care Med 2011;39(7):1683–91.

77. Malhotra S, Jordan D, Shortliffe E, et al. Workflow modeling in critical care: piecing together your own puzzle. J Biomed Inform 2007;40(2):81–92.

78. Laxmisan A, Hakimzada F, Sayan OR, et al. The multitasking clinician: decision-making and cognitive demand during and after team handoffs in emergency care. Int J Med Inform 2007;76(11–12):801–11.

79. Patel VL, Zhang J, Yoskowitz NA, et al. Translational cognition for decision support in critical care environments: a review. J Biomed Inform 2008;41(3):413–31.

80. Kanter RK. Would triage predictors perform better than first-come, first-served in pandemic ventilator allocation? Chest 2015;147(1):102–8.

81. Hick JL, O'laughlin DT. Concept of operations for triage of mechanical ventilation in an epidemic. Acad Emerg Med 2006;13(2):223–9.

82. King MA, Kissoon N. Triage during pandemics: difficult choices when business as usual is not an ethically defensible option. Crit Care Med 2016;44(9):1793–5.

83. Ashton-Cleary D, Tillyard A, Freeman N. Intensive care admission triage during a pandemic: a survey of the acceptability of triage tools. J Intensive Care Soc 2011; 12(3):180–6.

84. Vassallo J, Smith JE, Bruijns SR, et al. Major incident triage: a consensus based definition of the essential life-saving interventions during the definitive care phase of a major incident. Injury 2016;47(9):1898–902.

85. Antommaria AHM, Powell T, Miller JE, et al. Ethical issues in pediatric emergency mass critical care. Pediatr Crit Care Med 2011;12(6):S163–8.

86. Group UoTJCfBPIW. Stand on Guard for Thee. Ethical considerations in preparedness planning for pandemic influenza. Toronto: University of Toronto; 2005.

87. Ram-Tiktin E. Ethical considerations of triage following natural disasters: the IDF experience in Haiti as a case study. Bioethics 2017;31(6):467–75.

88. Biddison LD, Berkowitz KA, Courtney B, et al. Ethical considerations: care of the critically ill and injured during pandemics and disasters: CHEST consensus statement. Chest 2014;146(4 Suppl):e145S–55S.

89. Winsor S, Bensimon CM, Sibbald R, et al. Identifying prioritization criteria to supplement critical care triage protocols for the allocation of ventilators during a pandemic influenza. Healthc Q 2014;17(2):44–51.

90. Gostin LO, Hanfling D. National preparedness for a catastrophic emergency crisis standards of care. JAMA 2009;302(21):2365–6.

91. Powell T, Dan H, Gostin LO. Emergency preparedness and public health: the lessons of Hurricane Sandy. JAMA 2012;308(24):2569–70.

92. Courtney B, Hodge JG Jr, Toner ES, et al. Legal preparedness: care of the critically ill and injured during pandemics and disasters: CHEST consensus statement. Chest 2014;146(4 Suppl):e134S–44S.

93. Morton MJ, DeAugustinis ML, Velasquez CA, et al. Developments in surge research priorities: a systematic review of the literature following the Academic Emergency Medicine Consensus Conference, 2007-2015. Acad Emerg Med 2015;22(11):1235–52.

94. Morton B, Tang L, Gale R, et al. Performance of influenza-specific triage tools in an H1N1-positive cohort: P/F ratio better predicts the need for mechanical ventilation and critical care admission. Br J Anaesth 2015;114(6):927–33.

95. Adeniji KA, Cusack R. The Simple Triage Scoring System (STSS) successfully predicts mortality and critical care resource utilization in H1N1 pandemic flu: a retrospective analysis. Crit Care 2011;15(1):R39.

Natural Disasters

Jorge Hidalgo, MD, MACP, MCCM[a],*,
Amado Alejandro Baez, MD, MSc, MPH[b,c,1]

KEYWORDS

- Natural disaster • Classification of natural disasters • Preparedness • Hurricane
- Earthquake

KEY POINTS

- Natural disasters can cause a rupture of the daily routine with an essential impact on the local resources and the standard functionality of the population.
- It is critical that as health care personnel, we are familiar with different types of disasters and their plans of action.
- A fundamental part of our response is to be familiar with our hospital's plan of action and the role that we play in it.
- Intensive care units need to be involved in all preparedness efforts, so everyone can assess the strengths and weaknesses of our services; we also must be familiar with the intensive care evacuation plan.

INTRODUCTION

Natural disasters are unexpected predictable and unpredictable events that can have a severe impact in the population, with significant damage to infrastructure and important life and economic losses. Advances in technology have helped in the prediction of storms, hurricanes, and cyclones; however, a considerable amount of natural disasters can still present unexpectedly, such as earthquakes, volcano eruptions, and wildfires. In some instances there is a window of opportunity for warning but often this is short with catastrophic results, especially in those areas where the occurrence of a disaster is rare and the population is unprepared. From an organizational point of view, there is a need to make all necessary preparations, and this needs to be done collectively, with the involvement of the community and the health system, with the intensive care unit (ICU) necessarily being a part of all efforts to anticipate response and the potential for a possible evacuation.

The authors have no financial conflicts of interest to disclose.
[a] Karl Heusner Memorial Hospital, Princess Margaret Drive, PO Box 1355 883, Bellas Vista, Belize, Central America; [b] Department of Emergency Medicine/Center for Operational Medicine, Medical College of Georgia, Augusta University, 1120 15th St, Augusta, GA 30912, USA; [c] Universidad Nacional Pedro Henriquez Urena, Km 7 1/2, Avenida John F. Kennedy, Santo Domingo, Dominican Republic
[1] Dr A.A. Baez contributed equally to this article.
* Corresponding author.
E-mail address: jluishidalgo58@hotmail.com

In this article we review the most common natural disaster events; the magnitude, impact on the community, and vulnerability; immediate effects, including infrastructure damage and the threat to life; and how the health care system needs to be prepared and integrated with all the essential services of a community working to the maximum capacity. The community's capability and vulnerability and the effects of a disaster need to be revisited time to time in terms of resources and capacity of response. From a health care system standpoint, it is of the utmost importance that all necessary steps be implemented with time to prepare emergency systems and intensive care services as to how to respond and develop the strategies needed to be organized with an all-hazards approach. The main goal any health care–related disaster preparedness effort is to minimize the number of casualties and reduce suffering. It is important to mention that natural disasters can behave differently, and all preparedness and response efforts need to be flexible and dynamic with adaptability. In the case of critical care and ICU services, there needs to be an understanding of how to best deliver ethical but often unconventional care to optimize the greatest good delivered.

Natural Disasters

Natural disasters are complicated events. Preparation and an understanding of realistic capabilities of ICU units is paramount, including vulnerability assessment and the development of an all-hazards emergency management plan that integrates drills to better understand institutional response including the possibility of an evacuation plan.[1] Every disaster scenario is unique and presents new and unusual challenges to victims and rescue emergency personnel, challenging ICU capabilities. We need to analyze each disaster independently to recognize the distinctive features of the situation at hand. The classification of natural disasters is shown in **Box 1**.

Box 1
Classification of natural disasters

Geophysical	Hydrologic	Meteorologic	Climatologic
• Earthquake	• Flood	• Storm	• Extreme temperature
Ground shaking	1. General flood	1. Tropical cyclone	1. Heat wave
Tsunami	2. Flash flood	2. Extratropical	2. Cold wave
• Volcano	3. Storm surge/ coastal flood	Cyclone (winter storm)	Frost
Volcano eruption	• Mass movement (wet)	a. Convective storm	3. Extreme winter conditions
• Mass movement (dry)		Thunderstorm/ lightning	
1. Rockfall	1. Rockfall	Snowstorm/ blizzard	Snow pressure
2. Landslide	2. Landslide	Sandstorm/dust storm	Icing
Mudslide	Debris flood	Generic (severe) storm	Freezing rain
Lahar	3. Avalanche	Tornado	Debris avalanche
Debris flow	Snow avalanche	Orographic storm (strong winds)	• Drought
3. Avalanche	Debris avalanche	b. Local storm	• Wildfire
Snow avalanche	4. Subsidence		1. Forest fire
Debris avalanche	Sudden subsidence		2. Land fire
4. Subsidence	Long-lasting subsidence		
Sudden subsidence			
Long-lasting subsidence			

Certain disaster scenarios can follow general patterns and develop along similar paths. It is vital to appreciate these patterns to provide community planners and allied health professionals with a foundation to design a comprehensive emergency response plan.[1-3] A delicate balance must be maintained between learning from mistakes and lessons of the past and resisting the temptation of merely approaching "the way it has always been done."[4]

In planning, one needs to review how to organize the ICU disaster response. The first item is to make a diagnosis of resources, current critical care capacity, threat analysis, and how all of this will impact ICU care with an imperative need to meet with other clinical areas and services, such as the emergency department, hospital wards, and operating rooms, and integrate cohesively over a unified command structure. In general an emergency warning is usually available for the general population (**Fig. 1**).

Generally speaking, certain disaster types can lead to somewhat predictable injuries and illness patterns. This is an essential fact to keep in mind when planning an emergency response, taking stock of available medical supplies, or estimating the requirements of a population or geographic area.[3-6] It is critical, however, to be conscious that the injury and illness types are not exclusive to any one situation. Indeed, the sheer scale and complexity of a natural disaster may lead to many different smaller disaster situations, each one with its characteristics and challenges.[3,5-7] An example of a large-scale catastrophe causing many more minor emergencies situation is a large-scale flood, which in turn causes damage to a chemical factory, a landslide destroying several homes, drinking water reservoir contamination, and the collapse of buildings. As a basis for planning, it is important to consider the types of injuries most victims will incur to evaluate the immediate needs of the disaster response team.[8-10] We next cover specific natural disaster types and general items for which to anticipate and prepare. Some community response examples are shown in **Fig. 2**.

Hurricanes, Typhoons, and Cyclones

A powerful storm with violent winds (>74 mph) is what defines a hurricane, also known as a tropical cyclone in the Caribbean. The scientific community works hard to develop the necessary tools to predict significant disaster and with the technology

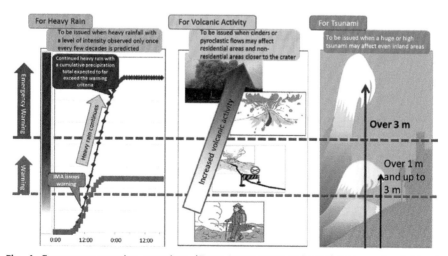

Fig. 1. Emergency warning overview. (*From* Japan Meteorological Agency: Available at: https://www.jma.go.jp/jma/en/Emergency_Warning/ew_index.html.)

Weather Warning/Advisory type							Municipal responses	Resident responses
Heavy rain		Storm	Storm surge	High waves	Heavy snow	Snowstorm		
Sediment incident	Inundation							
Emergency Warning (Significant likelihood of catastrophe) — Heavy rain Emergency Warning (sediment incident)	Heavy rain Emergency Warning (inundation)	Storm Emergency Warning	Storm surge Emergency Warning	High wave Emergency Warning	Heavy snow Emergency Warning	Snowstorm Emergency Warning	• Immediately urge residents to take all possible steps for self-protection • Alert residents to the issuance of an Emergency Warning and highlight the exceptionally dangerous situation	• Take immediate action for self-protection (head to an evacuation center, or if it is dangerous to go outside, evacuate to a safer place within the building)
Sediment Incident Alert							• Urge residents to evacuate • Issue evacuation advisories and orders to areas as necessary • Prepare for emergency response • Issue evacuation preparedness information to trigger evacuation of people requiring assistance • Establish evacuation centers • Disseminate Warnings to residents	• Start voluntary and early evacuation or follow evacuation advisories/orders • For Storm Warnings, evacuate to a safe place • Report abnormalities to municipalities and other authorities • Stay away from hazardous places • Prepare for evacuation
Warning (Chance of catastrophe) — Heavy rain Warning (sediment incident)	Heavy rain Warning (inundation)	Storm Warning	Storm surge Warning	High wave Warning	Heavy snow Warning	Snowstorm Warning		
Advisory (Possible development of serious adverse conditions) — Heavy rain Advisory		Gale Advisory	Storm surge Advisory	High waves Advisory	Heavy snow Advisory	Snowstorm Advisory	• Patrol areas requiring caution • Advise residents to pay attention • Monitor weather bulletins and information on rainfall conditions • Prepare to call out relevant officials	• Check emergency supplies • Check evacuation routes and centers • Check windows and storm shutters • Monitor weather bulletins on TV, radio and JMA's website

Fig. 2. Examples of municipal and resident responses to weather/advisories. (*From* Japan Meteorological Agency: Available at: https://www.jma.go.jp/jma/en/Emergency_Warning/ew_index.html.)

available it helps to predict significant storms and also anticipate the possible dimension of damage and destruction based on the assessment of trajectory and speed. In recent years there has been substantial and sustained population growth and along with that aggressive development of vulnerable coastal areas, which has led to an increase in hurricane-related deaths, injuries, and economic costs.[11–14] Hurricanes are called by other names depending on where they occur, such as typhoons in the Western Pacific Ocean and cyclones in the Indian Ocean. Hurricane consequences are divided based on the time and extension of the destruction.

Surge
Surge is defined as abnormal seawater level rise during a storm and caused primarily by a storm's winds pushing water inland. It is related to vital hurricane mortality.[15] The location of the coastline determines the amplitude of surge. Storm tide is illustrated in **Fig. 3**. These are essential factors to consider in hospital disaster preparedness, such as the impact of flash flooding on lower level floors, including the emergency department, and the location of power generators.

Winds
In a hurricane, the winds are a significant cause of mortality, and it helps to categorize the magnitude of anticipated destruction or damaged based on the speed of the winds. Classification of a hurricane is shown in **Table 1**.[16] One can experience significant property damage, flying objects, wind pressure, and objects can become airborne. Common injuries are those related to flying glass and other debris.

Tornadoes
A tornado is a violent, destructive rotating column of air extending from the base of a thunderstorm down to the ground. With tornados, there is the disadvantage of no warning, giving a community little time to prepare or seek shelter, and hence they see an increase in morbidity and mortality compared with other disasters. The related injuries are craniocerebral injury that can lead to immediate death or critical injury that requires admission to critical care services. Falling structures are responsible for crush injuries,

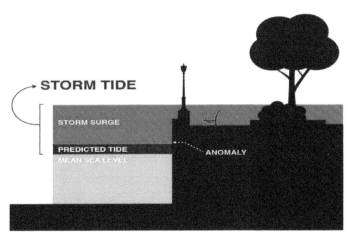

Fig. 3. Understanding storm tide. (*From* National Ocean Service. National Oceanic and Atmospheric Administration. Available at: https://oceanservice.noaa.gov/facts/stormsurge-stormtide.html.)

Table 1		
Saffir-Simpson hurricane wind scale		
Category	**Sustained Winds**	**Damage that is Expected Because of Hurricane Winds**
1	74–95 mph 64–82 kt 119–153 km/h	Very dangerous winds will produce some damage
2	96–110 mph 83–95 kt 154–177 km/h	Extremely dangerous winds will cause extensive damage
3 major	111–129 mph 96–112 kt 178–208 km/h	Devastating damage will occur
4 major	130–156 mph 113–136 kt 209–251 km/h	Catastrophic damage will occur
5 major	157 mph or higher 137 kt or higher 252 km/h or higher	Catastrophic damage will occur

(*From* National Hurricane Center, Available at: https://www.nhc.noaa.gov/aboutsshws.php.)

and fractures, contusions, abrasions, and soft tissue injuries that require transfer to an emergency room. The classification of tornados is shown in **Tables 2** and **3**.

Wound contamination and subsequent infection become an important factor in postoperative sepsis, leading to an increased need for aggressive wound care and surgical debridement. One-fifth of fracture injuries in the aftermath of a tornado is expected to be open, contributing to infection rates among patients.[17] Studies have shown that because of the proportion of projectile injuries, one-half to two-thirds of tornado victims who require surgery exhibit signs of early bacteremia and sepsis. A possible fatal outcome of sepsis is multiple organ failure.[3]

Floods

A flood is a general temporal condition of a partial or complete inundation. There are several types of floods resulting in long, short, or no warning with speed at the onset that is gradual or sudden. There is a seasonal pattern with significant effects related mainly to inundation and erosion, which can lead to community isolation and require a large-scale evacuation. The most important flood-related cause of mortality is drowning. In North America, floods account for more weather deaths than all other

Table 2		
Tornado Fujita scale (or F Scale) classification		
F-0	40–72 mph	Light damage
F-1	72–112 mph	Moderate damage
F-2	113–157 mph	Considerable damage
F-3	158–205 mph	Severe damage
F-4	206–260 mph	Devastating damage
F-5	261–318 mph	Violent damage

(National weather services. Available at: https://www.weather.gov/oun/tornadodata-okc-appendix.)

Table 3 Tornado enhanced Fujita scale		
Tornado Scale	Wind Speed	Level of Damage
EF0	65–85 mph	Light damage
EF1	86–109 mph	Moderate
EF2	110–137 mph	Considerable
EF3	138–167 mph	Severe
EF4	168–199 mph	Devastating
EF5	200–234 mph	Incredible

(National weather services. Available at: https://www.weather.gov/oun/tornadodata-okc-appendix.)

natural disasters, except for heat illnesses. The most significant number of deaths and injuries occur when there is little to no warning of an impending flood. This can happen in the case of flash flooding, the collapse of a dam, or from the action of a tidal wave as a result of a distant or suboceanic earthquake.[10] Most of the time, individuals underestimate the power of moving water, leading to what could have been many preventable deaths and injuries. In the best of times, it is complicated to estimate the average depth of opaque and fast-moving water; and it is next to impossible at dusk or in the middle of the night. It takes less than two feet of active moving water to float a big vehicle, such as a school bus, and only an average of 3 to 6 inches of fast active moving water to sweep a large man.[11]

The second flood-related cause of mortality is exposure to environmental elements, accounting for a large percentage of the deaths and critical serious lesions that happen during floods. In most cases, individuals who are caught in rising floodwaters wait for rescue in any refuge that is found including trees, inside their vehicles, and at the top of buildings. Depending on the extent of the flooding people may spend hours to days openly exposed to inclement weather, awaiting any rescue groups available.[12] The more the ambient temperature falls lower than 15°C, the greater the risk of accidental hypothermia.[3]

Landslide

Landslides are a type of "mass wasting," denoting any down-slope movement of soil and rock under the direct influence of gravity. In landslide the probability of warning varies, such as in an earthquake. There is some or no possibility of warning, a difference in the case of continuous rain. The speed of onset most times is rapid with significant damage to structures and systems (villages can be wholly swept away). Some secondary damage is related to the blockage of river flow, which can lead to flooding. Crops are affected. In some cases, the landslides are in combination with heavy rains and subsequent flooding and movements of debris. It can be difficult to access the affected areas, which can interfere with the rescue of victims, leading to a rehabilitation and recovery that is complex and expensive, and in some severe cases probably not possible.

Earthquakes

Earthquakes are a sudden and violent shaking of the earth's lithosphere and can cause major destruction. Important considerations when it comes to earthquakes are the lack of warning, speed of onset that often is sudden, and aftershocks. Some of the areas that are more susceptible to earthquake are well known, and most of the effects are from land movement, fracture, or slippage. With critical damage it can cause an important number of casualties because of the lack of warning. Large earthquakes are always followed by a series of aftershocks. These aftershocks have often slowed the pace of rescue missions, because they present significant threats to the safety of people. Thus, the establishment of emergency evacuation plans and safety protocols is imperative for conducting a compelling rescue mission. These aftershocks not only affect immediate operations but create a psychology of fear, especially when caring for victims, which warrants considerations for response and field hospital operations. Earthquake classification is shown in **Table 4**.

Mortality caused by crush injuries from falling objects is most frequently seen in earthquakes, with a considerable risk if indoors or in proximity to buildings or other structures. The risk of injury in the open is low.[4] Furthermore, injury severity is inversely related to epicenter distance to the earthquake. Injuries and deaths generally increase with the magnitude of the earthquake, increased ground motion, and structural damage.[7]

It is also noticed that trauma to the pelvis, thorax, and spine are seen when an earthquake happens during the night, most likely because victims are lying down in bed at the time of the disaster. These injuries commonly lead to severe internal organ injury, coinciding with bleeding. Lesions of the extremities with comorbid lacerations, severe external bleeding, and crush injuries including rhabdomyolysis and compartment syndrome are more commonly seen when the earthquake occurs during the daytime.[4]

Victims that have been trapped in fallen debris for hours or in some cases days run the risk of having infected wounds. Standard trauma procedures that need to be urgently addressed include amputations, vascular stabilization, fasciotomies, orthopedic stabilization, and debridement and/or dressing of open wounds. Patients with crush injuries also run a high risk of developing hypovolemic shock, hyperkalemia, and renal failure, and have an increased risk of fatal cardiac arrhythmia or myocardial infarction.[3] Although most earthquake-related trauma is a direct result of falling debris or collapsing structures, fire is another primary concern within the first golden 24 hours after the disaster. Depending on the size and extent of wildfires, burn injuries and respiratory problems caused by smoke inhalation can quickly become a significant strain

Table 4
Earthquake classification scales and damage observed

Richter Magnitude	Mercalli Intensity	Witness Observation
1–1.9	I	Microearthquakes, not felt or felt rarely.
2–2.9	I-II	Felt slightly for some people. No damage to buildings.
3–3.9	II-IV	Often felt by people. Infrequently causes injuries.
4–4.9	VI-VI	Noticeable. Felt by most people in the affected areas.
5–5.9	VI-VII-	Can cause damage of varying severity, depends on the quality of the construction.
6–6.9	VIII-X	Damage to a moderate number of well-built structures in populated areas.
7–7.9	X or greater	Cause damage to most buildings.
8–8.9	X or greater	Major damage.
9 or greater	X or greater	At or near to total destruction.

(*Adapted from* USGS. Available at: https://earthquake.usgs.gov/learn/topics/mag_vs_int.php.)

on the medical system after an earthquake.[3] Some measures that the general popu-lation can take are shown in **Fig. 4**.

Tsunami

A tsunami is a long high sea wave caused by an earthquake, submarine landslide, or other disturbance; it is destructive with high waves. The velocity depends on the depth of the water where the seismic problem originated with a variable speed of onset. An alert time can sometimes be granted depending on the monitoring and origin of the triggering event. Wave heights can reach up to 30 m and be preceded by a marked recession of average water level before the arrival of the wave that results in a massive ongoing tide, followed by the tsunami wave. The health impact can cause immediate trauma and drowning, but later can cause saltwater contamination of the soil and crops and damage to water supplies, and essential flooding and significant damage to infrastructure. All efforts are needed to warn the population, prepare threatened communities for evacuation with effective time-scale to high ground areas, and with a recovery phase that could be extensive and costly. Tsunami warning example is shown in **Fig. 5**.

Drought

Drought is a natural disaster that is below average and leads to a period of extensive abnormally low rainfall, leading to a shortage of water. The areas that are susceptible to drought are usually known beforehand, which allows for a potential warning period. Drought can have a significant impact on the availability of food because it impacts agriculture and livestock resources. The response requirements may be extensive and prolonged and can undermine self-reliance of affected communities, leading to less common nonacute problems than those seen the ICU setting, but still stressing the local health system.

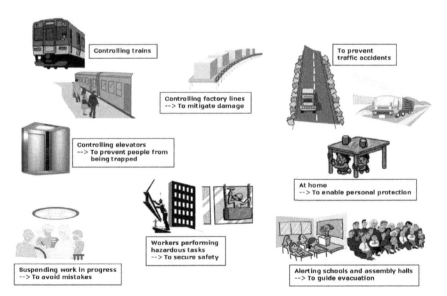

Fig. 4. Examples of response to an earthquake early warning. (*From* Japan Meteorological Agency. Available at: https://www.jma.go.jp/jma/en/Activities/eew2.html.)

Estimated maximum tsunami height		Action to be taken	Expected damage
Quantitative expression	For huge earthquakes		

			Action to be taken	Expected damage
Major Tsunami Warning	**over 10 m** (10 m < height)		Evacuate from coastal or river areas immediately to safer places such as high ground or a tsunami evacuation building. Tsunami waves are expected to hit repeatedly. Do not leave the evacuation location until Tsunami Warnings are cleared. *Keep evacuating to higher and higher ground wherever possible!* Educational video "Escape the Tsunami" (JMA)	Wooden structures are expected to be completely destroyed and/or washed away; anybody exposed will be caught in tsunami currents. (Most wooden structures washed away due to the tsunami in 2011)
	10 m (5m < height ≤ 10m)	Huge		
	5m (3 m < height ≤ 5 m)			
Tsunami Warning	**3m** (1 m < height ≤ 3 m)	High		Tsunami waves will hit, causing damage to low-lying areas. Buildings will be flooded and anybody exposed will be caught in tsunami currents. Toyokoro-cho (2003)
Tsunami Advisory	**1m** (20 cm ≤ height ≤ 1 m)	(N/A)	Get out of the water and leave coastal areas immediately. Do not engage in fishing or swimming activities until Advisories are cleared.	Anybody exposed will be caught in a strong tsunami currents in the sea. Fish farming facilities will be washed away and small vessels may capsize.

Fig. 5. Tsunami warning/advisory categories and action to be taken. (1) Tsunamis may hit before warnings are issued if the source region is near the coast. Be sure to evacuate when shaking occurs. (2) Tsunami heights may exceed estimations because of coastal topography and other factors in some regions. Evacuate to higher ground. (3) Tsunami forecasts (slight sea level change) are issued if the estimated tsunami height is less than 20 cm and no damage is expected, or if slight sea level changes are expected after tsunami advisories are cleared. (*From* Japan Meteorological Agency. Available at: https://www.jma.go.jp/jma/en/Emergency_Warning/ew_index.html.)

Fires

In general, areas prone to bushfires are known; they tend to occur seasonally and are well defined. The speed of onset can vary and is affected by weather, temperature, and wind speed, which can spread fiery fragments to other areas starting new fires, also known as "spotting." Approximately 90% of forest fires in the United States are caused by human action; natural forest fires most often occur because of lightning strikes in dry and windy conditions. The most significant health impact of a forest fire is the effect on the surrounding air quality. Because of favorable local conditions, many smaller fires can contribute to the poor air quality of one particular area. At best, the buildup of smoke and pollutants in the air decreases visibility, and at worst, it can create new respiratory problems or can exacerbate existing conditions.[6] Burn injuries from forest fires are rare but not unheard of; they are most likely associated with firefighters who are commonly called on to be nearby massive and unpredictable fires. Depending on the existing wind condition, forest fires can spread rapidly and change direction quickly, which can lead to entrapment of firefighters and less commonly, private citizens.[6]

Occasionally, within the context of vast forest fires animal attacks and/or bites also increase. Depending on the proximity of a wildfire to a community, a good amount of the wild animals who have been forced to abandoned their habitat often come into contact with humans.[8] This phenomenon, which is also seen in massive floods, can lead not only to trauma from animal attacks but more commonly increased infections (infection passed from animals to humans).[9] Great fires that range through urban areas are less common in developed countries because of the advent of trained and equipped personal. However, large-scale urban fires are always possible in the developing world and secondary to other natural disasters. Injuries in a large-scale urban fire are frequently burn injuries and deaths associated with asphyxiation. Common complications of burn injuries include major loss of fluids, which leads to hypovolemic shock and massive infections and sepsis.

Heat Waves

Heat waves are known as the silent disaster. Between 1979 and 1999, more than 8000 people in the United States died from a hyperthermic illness. This represents more deaths than earthquakes and other common natural catastrophes combined. Consequences of health effects in a heat wave usually are first noticeable among vulnerable populations within an affected area. People with a medical problem, the elderly, and the very young are all especially susceptible to heat stress, and a patient can easily go from heat exhaustion to potentially fatal heat stroke.[13] However, everybody is susceptible to heat illness if the proper precautions are not taken.

One can prevent heat illnesses by taking simple measures, such as shortening the length of time spent exposed to high temperatures. Another critical aspect of preventative measures is to maintain fluid body status by drinking enough liquids and abstaining from alcoholic and energetic beverages. Treatment of advanced stages of heat stroke includes rapid cooling of the body and urgent fluid and electrolyte replacement. When cooling is initiated, the core body temperature must be monitored to guard against rebound hyperthermia or inadvertent hypothermia.[13] The mortality rate for heat stroke depends on the duration and severity of the hyperthermia and access to early health assistance.

Winter Storms

The immediate effect of winter storms, depending on severity, is in disruption of traffic patterns and a sharp spike in automobile accidents. Trauma from traffic collisions can vary from an orthopedic injury, severe vascular compromise, to life-threatening bruising to the thorax and abdomen. Head injuries, fractures, and bruising are also provoked by falls in icy walking conditions and are more common among the elderly.[18] Exposure to the elements is also of major concern in a winter storm. Individuals may incur frostbite from exposure to cold for an extended period of time and in severe cases may require amputation.

Because power lines and telephone systems are commonly disrupted in a severe winter storm, death from carbon monoxide poisoning and hypothermia is also a considerable concern because individuals frequently use inappropriate heaters indoors to stay warm.[19] Additionally, death and injury from fires are common in winter storms because individuals leave candles, fireplaces, and heaters burning throughout the night for use as either heat and light.[19] Furthermore, as previously sedentary individuals venture outside to make repairs or clear snow during winter storms, there is an increase in acute coronary syndrome.

Volcanoes

Volcanic activity can be monitored, and most eruptions are predicted. The volcanic eruption and blast can cause significant destruction of nearby structures, and the surrounding environment becomes almost immediately threatening to life and health as airborne pollutants are ejected into the atmosphere. Like smoke from massive forest fires, the airborne pollutants may cause new respiratory diseases or exacerbate existing conditions. With volcanoes, however, the sheer magnitude of an important eruption can fill the atmosphere with an incredible amount of ash and lethal gases. The ash in its airborne form can cause damage to aircraft by seeping into the engines. If caught within proximity of an eruption, even individuals with no respiratory illnesses find it hard to breathe. Common effects of toxic volcanic gases, such as carbon dioxide, carbon monoxide, and sulfuric acid, include acute respiratory distress syndrome (including pulmonary edema), conjunctivitis, arthralgias, muscle weakness, and cutaneous bullae.[3] Burns caused by superheated steam or as a result of secondary fires started by the eruption are also common. In many instances mudslides occur in conjunction with volcanic eruptions as the topographic contour or the hillside rapidly changes. Landslides, which are commonly seen as flooding situations, can lead to asphyxiation crushing injuries, severe internal bleeding, and multiple organ dysfunction syndrome. What is challenging is access to the site of the eruption and the timing and accurate evacuation decision, especially if there have been previous false alarms. Volcanic warning systems are shown in **Figs. 6** and **7**.

NATURAL DISASTER AFTERMATH

Apart from the immediate trauma and injuries suffered by victims of natural disasters, studies have shown that several secondary medical conditions increase in incidence in the critical hours and days after, during the assessment and recovery period. In many cases, these secondary medical problems are attributed, at least in part, to the immense stress placed on individuals during a disaster situation. Disaster stress varies from person to person, and each person is vulnerable to different types and levels. It has also been suggested that "fight or flight," a normal physiologic response initiated during times of perceived personal danger like those seen in natural disasters (eg, earthquake), is contributory to postcatastrophe acute myocardial infarctions. The fight or flight response, considered as a systemic sympathetic nervous

Classification	Name of Warning with targeted area	Targeted area	Level	Keyword	Expected volcanic activity	Action to be taken by residents	Action to be taken by climbers
Emergency Warning	Volcanic Warning (residential areas[a]) (a.k.a. Residential-area Warning)	Residential areas[a] and non-residential areas nearer the crater	5	Evacuate	Eruption or imminent eruption that may cause serious damage in residential and non-residential areas nearer the crater	Evacuate from the danger zone. (Targeted areas and evacuation measures are determined in line with current volcanic activity.)	
			4	Prepare to evacuate	Possibility or increasing possibility of eruption that may cause serious damage in residential and non-residential areas nearer the crater	Prepare to evacuate from alert areas. Have disabled people evacuate. (Target areas and evacuation measures are determined in line with current volcanic activity.)	
Warning	Volcanic Warning (near the crater) (a.k.a. Near-crater Warning)	Non-residential areas near the crater	3	Do not approach the volcano	Eruption or possibility of eruption that may severely affect places near residential areas (possible threat to life in such areas)	Stand by and pay attention to changes in volcanic activity. Have disabled people prepare to evacuate in line with current volcanic activity.	Refrain from entering the danger zone. (Targeted areas are determined in line with current volcanic activity.)
		Around the crater	2	Do not approach the crater	Eruption or possibility of eruption that may affect areas near the crater (possible threat to life in such areas)	No action required	Refrain from approaching the crater. (Targeted areas around the crater are determined in line with current volcanic activity.)
Forecast	N/A	Inside the crater	1	Potential for increased activity	Calm: Possibility of volcanic ash emissions or other related phenomena in the crater (possible threat to life in the crater)		No restrictions (In some cases, it may be necessary to refrain from approaching the crater.)

Fig. 6. Volcanic warning system (for volcanoes where volcanic alert levels are applied). [a] When residential areas are not defined, "residential areas" is replaced with "foot-of-mountain areas." (*From* Japan Meteorological Agency. Available at: https://www.data.jma.go.jp/svd/vois/data/tokyo/STOCK/kaisetsu/English/level.html.)

Classification	Name of Warning with targeted area	Targeted area	Keyword	Expected volcanic activity
Emergency Warning	Volcanic Warning (residential areas[a]) (a.k.a. Residential-area Warning)	Residential areas[a] and non-residential areas nearer the crater	Extreme caution advised in residential areas[a] and non-residential areas nearer the crater	Eruption or possibility of eruption that may cause serious damage in residential areas[a] and non-residential areas nearer the crater
Warning	Volcanic Warning (near the crater) (a.k.a. Near-crater Warning)	Non-residential areas near the crater	Caution advised in non-residential areas near the crater	Eruption or possibility of eruption that may severely affect places near residential areas (possible threat to life in such areas)
		Around the crater	Caution advised around the crater	Eruption or possibility of eruption that may affect areas near the crater (possible threat to life in such areas)
Forecast	N/A	Inside the crater	Potential for increased activity	Calm: Volcanic ash emissions or other related phenomena may occur in the crater (possible threat to life in the crater)

Fig. 7. Volcanic warning system (for volcanoes where volcanic alert levels are NOT applied). [a] When residential areas are not defined, "residential areas" is replaced with "foot-of-mountain areas." (*From* Japan Meteorological Agency. Available at: https://www.data.jma.go.jp/svd/vois/data/tokyo/STOCK/kaisetsu/English/level.html.)

system response activation, leads to an increased vulnerability to myocardial infarctions in individuals with preexisting heart disease.[16–18] Along with outright heart attacks, other coronary events are seen after natural disasters, such as unstable angina and potentially fatal arrhythmias. In many instances, the effect of the increased stress load is compounded with the interruption of regular medical services for preexisting conditions, such as asthma, chronic obstructive pulmonary disease, and diabetes.

Allergies and asthma are aggravated after a natural disaster. This is especially true in the case of large-scale ejection of pollutants into the atmosphere, as with a volcanic eruption or wildfire. This seems to be limited to those with preexisting asthmatic or bronchial conditions and heavily exposed rescue and recovery workers.[16–18] In many studies, there was not much description of *de novo* respiratory conditions among the general populace who received minimal to average amount of exposure to the airborne irritants.[16] Furthermore, it has been found that in the immediate aftermath of some disasters, the actual occurrence of severe asthmatic or allergic attacks decreased.[16]

Disaster stress has also been attributed to making current disease processes worse and reducing victims' abilities to fight off infection. A study of patients with rheumatoid arthritis showed that after an earthquake, the incidence of rheumatoid arthritis activity (pain, stiffness, and swelling) increases dramatically.[20,21] It has also been shown that because of the frequent occurrence of dehydration, malnutrition, breakdown of public health safeguards, and stress and anxiety in the aftermath of natural disaster, an individual is more prone to severe infection from a familiar vector, including disease vectors.[21]

In many cases, the stress and impact on a victim's health take a while to surface. This is common with the psychological implications of catastrophes. In the weeks and months following catastrophic events, many patients suffer from such mental disorders as post-traumatic stress disorder or generalized anxiety disorder.[22] In many instances, hallucinations, flashbacks, night terrors, sudden phobias, grief, depression, guilt, insomnia, and loss of appetite are some of the symptoms and signs perceived by victims.[21,22] It is common for many behavioral responses to disaster and catastrophic events to remain subtly buried within a victim's coping mechanisms, and seen only under close observation of critical health-related habits, such as sleeping, eating, smoking, or alcohol intake. Psychological recovery from lapses in mental health, related or seen on natural disasters, is dependent on the timely recognition of fainting and access to the necessary resources that are used to promote healing.

As populations rise in high-risk areas, the potential for mass casualty natural disasters also rises. In the event of a catastrophe with numerous victims, the sheer volume would overload local response mechanisms. This would compound any existing stresses that surviving victims would face after an emergency. Scarce essential resources would now have to be shared with a higher number of victims. Volunteers and health professionals would have limited time.[1] Generally, the severity of secondary medical problems, many of which are in part attributed to stress, is directly dependent on the disaster type, the size of the disaster, and the community's ability to cope with and recover from the massive destruction.

DISRUPTION OF THE INITIAL EMERGENCY RESPONSE: THE RESCUE STAGE

In the hours following a significant natural disaster, the immediate rescue effort originates from the affected community itself. Local resources are quickly recruited and reorganized to suit the apparent needs at hand. In many instances, this is done on a case-by-case basis, and medical response measures may be initiated before the complete picture is considered. Within the first 24 hours, the priority remains to ensure that the most critically ill and accessible patients receive the proper medical attention and care. However, with many natural disasters, the situation is further complicated by the massive disruption of critical infrastructure, which prevents an appropriately organized and comprehensive medical response.

Health insurance may broadly be defined as "traditional lifeline systems within a given community or geographic area." Some systems contribute directly to community health, such as hospitals, clinics, emergency response units, and water treatment plants. Other methods, such as shelter, power, fuel, and communication, are not directly labeled as "medical care systems," but still contribute to the affected victims and public health.[21]

In the worst-case scenario, the core of the health infrastructure, the hospital, could be disrupted. A review of many natural disasters in the United States revealed that damage or collapse of a hospital is not often seen. Many of the disaster response protocols redesigned in the 1970s account for this possibility, even though the loss of power or water is more common than structural damage. Hence, most hospitals in North America are equipped with at least one, if not two, backup systems to ensure that a moderate degree of operability can occur in even the worst of situations (although in severe disasters even backup systems have been known to fail).[18] However, the situation is vastly different in developing countries. In many underdeveloped emergency care systems, energy failure or even structural damage are a real possibility in a severe disaster. In many cases, hospitals and clinics do not serve as additional disaster protection over the rest of the community, leaving the area vulnerable to a significant catastrophe.[22]

A powerful natural disaster may also impact directly other medical resources, such as fire trucks and ambulance vehicles. Damage to emergency vehicles is most critical in the early stages of the rescue operation because many victims seek transportation to medical centers. However, studies have shown that in a major disaster, many victims are brought to medical centers in taxis and private vehicles. Thus, damage or destruction of ambulances would acutely affect the critically ill patients who require specialized care at the scene or those in need of specialized medical attention.[22] Disruption of transportation routes also interferes with the initial medical emergency response. Roads, bridges, and tunnels can be damaged in natural disasters. Inclement weather from hurricanes, cyclones, or tornadoes makes impossible any attempt of victims to be rescue by helicopters and "medevac" aircraft. Just as emergency vehicles are prevented from reaching critically ill victims, patients in private vehicles are equally prevented from reaching hospitals and clinics.

Just as hospitals and emergency vehicles are vulnerable or destroyed by a natural disaster, so are medical supply depots and storage facilities. The damage or destruction of critical medical stores carrying medications, dressings, intravenous lines, and so forth can compound an already desperate situation. In the aftermath of any disaster, medical facilities require additional supplies in response to the increase in admission. The medical system's ability to provide care is surpassed in the event of natural disaster. A specific natural disaster may also require specialized supplies to treat the presenting specific injury patterns.[18] In some instances, the lack of appropriate medical supplies may contribute to a "secondary disaster" whereby victims who would have survived with medical care with time succumb to their injuries.

Furthermore, in natural disasters, where the type of lesion and loss of life are widespread, immediate medical care may be prevented by disaster planning that requires off-duty health workers be called in the event of a significant catastrophe. A prevailing assumption is that a medical facility may double or even triple its available workforce by activating off-duty personnel. In large-scale disasters, however, this is probably not the case. A review of medical practices after Taiwan Chi-Chi earthquake in 1999 shows that much medical personnel will only respond to the community after their own family's safety and well-being are ensured.[23,24] Combined with the loss or injury of other health care professionals, authorities in Taiwan faced a medical workforce of half the predicted size. Finally, because many physicians and nurses were "off-shift" at the time of the disaster they were prevented from reaching hospitals and clinics because of disrupted transportation systems.

A sign of a sophisticated emergency care system is the specific development of disaster protocols and medical subspecialties, such as trauma medicine, to deal with disaster injuries and challenges. Within the context of developed emergency planning, large tertiary hospitals take a central role in providing care for victims and even work as central points of organization for the community as a whole. Commonly, hospitals are structurally reinforced with the forethought of the role that they will play in the disaster recovery operation. With underdeveloped emergency care systems common in developing countries, medical care in a disaster situation is usually given by physicians and health care workers with no specific training in emergency medicine. In these circumstances, there is often a diffuse response to the disaster with no centralized point of the organization.[23]

SUMMARY

Natural disasters are complex and of diverse categories and impact. Over the past decade, significant attention has focused on preparing the health care system to handle disasters. ICU preparations are critical to any community's response because a large number of patients may be critically ill, and natural disasters happen at a significant rate.

Planning needs to have an all-hazards approach and be able to develop processes that enable the expansion of ICU capacity, and adapt standard of care in the likely event that a natural disaster increases the number of critically ill patients stressing already frail ICU systems.

Intensive care and critical care services are disrupted and overwhelmed significantly during the aftermath of a national disaster. Both acute and nonacute, traumatic and nontraumatic problems and illness can complicate the ICU operations of the affected community. A systematic evaluation and approach can result in mitigating consequences, with an essential focus on preparedness and integration of ICUs within the system. For an optimal health care response, it is imperative to understand regional and site-specific ICU capabilities and identify potential sites that in the event of a hospital evacuation, can adequately accommodate patients and personal.

REFERENCES

1. Novajan M, Salehi OB. Conceptual change of disaster management models: a thematic analysis. Jamba 2018;10(1):451.
2. Abbot P. Natural disaster. New York: Mc Graw Hill education, Tenth Edition Penn Plaza; 2017.
3. Scott Z, Wooster K, Few R, et al. Monitoring and evaluating a disaster risk management capacity. Disaster Prev Manag 2016;25(3):412–22.
4. Alexander DE. The game changes: disaster prevention and management after a quarter of century. Disaster Prev Manag 2016;25(1):2–10.
5. Saldaña-Zorrilla SO. Assessment of disaster risk management in Mexico. Disaster Prev Manag 2015;24(2):230–48.
6. Van der Waldt G. Disaster risk management: disciplinary status and prospects for a unifying theory. Journal of Disaster Risk Studies 2013.
7. Shi P, Xu W, et al. Developing disaster risk science, discussion on the disaster reduction implementation science. Natural Disaster Science 2011.
8. Zimmerman M, Stössel F. Disaster risk reduction in international cooperation: Switzerland contribution to the protection of lives and livelihoods. Berne (Switzerland): Swiss agency for development and collaboration; 2011.
9. Mohapatra R. Community based planning in post-disaster reconstruction: a case study of tsunami affected fishing communities in Tamil Nadu Coast of India. UW-Space; 2009.
10. Bass S, Ramasamy S, de Pryck JD, et al. Disaster risk management system analysis: A guide book. Rome (Italy): Food and Agriculture Organization of the United Nations; 2008.
11. Australian Development Gateway: Disaster risk cycle. Document. 2008.
12. Nick Carter W. Disaster management. Mandaluyong city (The Philippines): Asian development bank; 2008.
13. Moe TL, Pathranarakul P. An integrated approach to natural disaster management: Public project management and its critical success factors. Disaster Prev Manag 2006;15(3):396–413.

14. Ashgar S, Alahakoon D, Churilov L. A comprehensive conceptual model for disaster management. Journal of Humanitarian Assistance 2006.
15. Asgary A. Theorizing disaster and emergency management. In: Raj Kumar C, Srivastava DK, editors. Tsunami and disaster management: law and governance. Hong Kong: Sweet & Maxwell Asia; 2006.
16. Manitoba Health Disaster Management. Disaster management model for the health sector. Guideline for program development. Manitoba (Canada): Government of Manitoba; 2005.
17. Cannon, T. At risk: natural hazards, people vulnerability, and disaster. Paper presented at CENAT conference. Ticino, Switzerland, November 28–December 3, 2004.
18. Asian Disaster Preparedness Centre (ADPC). Community Based Disaster Management (CBDM): Trainer's guide, Module 4: Disaster management. Bangkok (Thailand): Asian Disaster Preparedness Centre; 2000.
19. Ice Storm '98 – A Case Study In Response (Kingston – Brockville) Queen's University – Human Resources Development Canada – Emergency Preparedness Canada.
20. Lin LY, Wu CC, Liu YB, et al. Derangement of heart rate variability during a catastrophic earthquake: a possible mechanism for increased heart attacks. Pacing Clin Electrophysiol 2001;24(11):1596–601.
21. Bernstein RS, Baxter PJ, Falk H, et al. Immediate public health concerns and actions during volcanic eruptions: lessons from the Mount St. Helens eruptions, May 18–October 18, 1980. Am J Public Health 1986;76(3 Suppl):25–37.
22. Bradshaw L, Fishwick D, Kep T, et al. Under the volcano: fire, ash and asthma. N Z Med J 1997;110(1040):90–1.
23. Auf der Heide E. The apathy factor. Disaster response: principles of preparation and coordination. St. Louis: Mosby; 1989.
24. Blankie P, Cannon T, Davis I, et al. At risk: natural hazards, people's vulnerability. London: Routledge; 1994.

Intensive Care Unit Preparedness During Pandemics and Other Biological Threats

Ryan C. Maves, MD*, Christina M. Jamros, DO[1],
Alfred G. Smith, DO[1]

KEYWORDS

- Pandemic • Influenza • Disaster preparedness

KEY POINTS

- In a globalized world where epidemics and pandemics are increasingly common, hospital preparation requires early planning.
- Infection prevention controls are critical during pandemics to reduce the risk to staff and other patients.
- In an emergency, ICU capacity may be increased by utilizing alternate hospital sites and non-ICU staff under the supervision of trained critical care personnel.
- Community engagement during a pandemic is important, to reduce alarm and also to ensure equitable distribution of limited resources.

INTRODUCTION

Outbreaks of infectious disease pose unique challenges for hospitals and intensive care units (ICUs). In the twentieth century, the polio pandemic led to the development of mechanical ventilation and was a major driver for the first units devoted to the care of patients with respiratory failure. The 2009 to 2010 H1N1 influenza pandemic, with

Disclosure: The authors have no financial conflicts of interest to disclose. The authors are US military service members. This work was prepared as part of their official duties. Title 17 U.S C. §105 provides that "Copyright protection under this title is not available for any work of the United States Government." Title 17 U.S C. §101 defines a US Government work as a work prepared by a military service member or employee of the US Government as part of that person's official duties. The views expressed in this article are those of the authors and do not necessarily reflect the official policy or position of the Departments of the Navy, the Department of Defense, nor the US Government.
Division of Infectious Diseases, Department of Internal Medicine, Naval Medical Center, 34800 Bob Wilson Drive, San Diego, CA 92134, USA
[1] These authors contributed equally to this article.
* Corresponding author.
E-mail address: ryan.c.maves.mil@mail.mil

previously healthy victims suffering from severe respiratory failure and refractory hypoxemia, helped drive the expansion of extracorporeal membrane oxygenation (ECMO) from an infrequently used salvage therapy to a major critical care intervention. Outbreaks of severe acute respiratory syndrome-associated coronavirus (SARS-CoV) disease in 2001 to 2002 and the 2013 to 2014 West African Ebola epidemic showed the risks of highly contagious disease to clinical staff and the potential of infectious diseases to spread quickly between continents.

Although sometimes used interchangeably, the differences between the terms "outbreak," "epidemic," and "pandemic" are primarily ones of scale. *Outbreaks* are local increases in disease incidence that may place strain on a single hospital or several hospitals in a region. In industrialized countries, the impact of outbreaks on critical care resources may be limited because of the availability of patient transfer to other facilities. *Epidemics* are similar to outbreaks in that they refer to an often sudden increase in the rate of a disease in a geographic area, but the common usage of the word "epidemic" implies a larger geographic area than an outbreak, with a greater potential impact on health care resources. A *pandemic* is an epidemic that affects multiple areas of the world; in the case of influenza, a pandemic is formally defined by the World Health Organization (WHO) as an epidemic occurring in at least 2 different nations in 2 different WHO regions.

The potential infectious threats to a hospital and its associated ICUs are numerous and varied, including antimicrobial-resistant pathogens, nosocomial infections, and common and predictable dangers such as seasonal influenza. It is not hyperbole to describe carbapenem-resistant Enterobacteriaceae as a pandemic threat, for example. These sorts of infections, however, place gradual strains on hospital systems and only rarely cause acute disasters.

The sorts of infections most likely to require a disaster-level response for ICUs in industrialized settings are respiratory viruses, specifically influenza, although coronaviruses have produced similar sorts of outbreaks with SARS-CoV and the more recent Middle Eastern Respiratory syndrome-associated coronavirus (MERS-CoV). Limitations in public health infrastructure in resource-constrained regions, such as reliable, clean water and vector control, may lead to epidemics of virulent but less-contagious pathogens such as cholera; natural disasters may directly cause or exacerbate such epidemics, as in Haiti following the January 2010 earthquake.

Hemorrhagic fever viruses have led to epidemics with global pandemic potential, as dramatically demonstrated by Ebola and related viruses. The unique infection prevention requirements, the intensity of staffing, and sophisticated training required for the care of viral hemorrhagic fevers mean that a small number of patients can easily overwhelm a health system.

For purposes of planning, the types of infectious diseases that are most likely to be implicated in disaster share certain key characteristics:

Virulence

A significant proportion of infected patients need to be at risk for organ failure and death. This proportion may be a minority of affected patients, but the risk of severe disease must be substantial and may not necessarily impact groups who are at "typical" risk for critical illness (eg, the elderly and immunocompromised).

Contagiousness

There may be a high risk of infection following exposure to an ill patient. Alongside this risk of transmission, the population at risk of exposure should generally lack immunity to the infecting pathogen. If a given epidemic pathogen is not especially contagious (ie, cholera), then it may result from an exposure that is difficult to avoid, such as widespread contamination of drinking water.

Although history provides numerous examples of public health emergencies due to infection, the 2003 outbreak of SARS-CoV, the 2009 to 2010 influenza A(H1N1) pandemic, and the limited number of Western patients infected with Ebola virus in 2014 to 2015 serve as a useful basis for future hospital and ICU-based planning.

Severe acute respiratory syndrome-associated coronavirus outbreaks, 2003

In February 2003, 300 people in the Guangdong Province of China were reported as suffering from a novel and severe respiratory illness, with 5 confirmed deaths at the time.[1,2] The following month, 11 health care workers (HCWs) were diagnosed with what was later named by the WHO as SARS—a coronavirus of presumably zoonotic origin.[1,3,4] A physician from Guangdong, not previously known to be infected with SARS, subsequently traveled to Hong Kong, leading to infection of several other visitors to the hotel in which he was staying.[3] These newly infected individuals then traveled via airplane, spreading the virus to Vietnam, Singapore, Ireland, Canada, and the United States.

The bulk of SARS cases occurred in eastern Asia, although 33 cases and 1 death were identified in Europe, 29 cases and no deaths in the United States, and 251 total cases with 43 deaths in Canada. Transmission and subsequent infection rates were high following exposure to patients who were infected with SARS, with up to 60% of exposed nurses in a Toronto hospital subsequently falling ill before the imposition of effective controls.[5] Among hospitalized patients, 10% to 20% progressed to hypoxemic respiratory failure requiring mechanical ventilation.[6,7] By July 2003, the outbreak had peaked with a total of 8096 documented infections with 774 deaths (case-fatality rate 9.6%).[3,8]

Throughout the outbreak, case identification and early management were limited by the nonspecific initial symptoms of SARS, with a respiratory viral prodrome progressing to fulminant disease that could quickly overwhelm a smaller community hospital with limited resources and staff.[9] Many hospitals lacked contingency plans for surge capacity, patient transfer, or sufficient numbers of trained staff. In addition, initial government delays in notifying the general public about the potential pandemic spread of this novel virus prevented hospitals from implementing proper infection control procedures, contributing to a disproportionate number of HCWs becoming infected with SARS. Similarly, an early lack of infection prevention protocols led to many of the earlier patients being assigned to rooms alongside uninfected patients, further increasing the spread of disease.[10] Although the primary outbreak peaked in May 2003, delayed secondary outbreaks were reported into June and July, in part due to relaxed infection control practices later in the epidemic.[11]

Influenza A(H1N1) pandemic, 2009 to 2010

Critical care services were challenged worldwide during the novel 2009 influenza A (H1N1) pandemic. The first cases emerged in the southwestern United States and Mexico in early 2009.[12] By late April 2009, reported cases of A(H1N1) had spread across North America and worldwide. By August 2010, when the pandemic had run its course, influenza had caused approximately 300,000 deaths worldwide, of which 200,000 were due to respiratory failure. Unlike typical influenza seasons, higher mortality was documented among children, young adults, and pregnant women.[13]

In Mexico City alone, 58 of 899 patients (6.5%) with influenza A(H1N1) hospitalized at 6 hospitals between March and June 2009 required critical care admission, a significant burden in facilities who averaged only 16 ICU beds per hospital.[12] In that setting, over a strained hospital system and delays in admission because of ICU over-crowding, there was an overall 60-day mortality of 41% of critically ill patients and an increased risk of death in critically ill patients receiving care outside of the ICU.

Even in higher-resource settings, ICU capacity was strained. Australia and New Zealand reported an 8-fold increase in influenza incidence during the southern hemi-spheric winter, compared with the same period in the United States.[14] In a cohort study of all ICUs in Australia and New Zealand from June through August 2009, 5.2% of ICU bed-days were from patients with 2009 H1N1 influenza and reached a peak percentage of ICU bed occupancy of 8.9% to 19.0%. The most significant effect on ICU resource consumption occurred 4 to 6 weeks after the first confirmed winter ICU admission, with extra workload lasting several weeks.[14]

In Canada, a prospective observational study of 38 adult and pediatric ICUs evalu-ated 168 critically ill patients infected with A(H1N1), of whom 136 patients (81.0%) required mechanical ventilation for a median duration of 12 days. Additional lung rescue therapies included neuromuscular blockade (28% of patients), inhaled nitric oxide (13.7%), high-frequency oscillatory ventilation (11.9%), ECMO (4.2%), and prone positioning ventilation (3.0%).[15] Ninety-day mortality in this cohort was 17.3%, less than in Mexico City, but still substantial despite the increased resources that could be brought to bear.

West Africa Ebola virus disease epidemic, 2014 to 2016

In March 2014, the Ministries of Health in the West African nations of Guinea and Liberia reported outbreaks of Ebola virus disease (EVD) that rapidly spread to nearby countries and overseas. The resulting EVD epidemic affected over 28,000 persons in Guinea, Liberia, and Sierra Leone, in addition to smaller case numbers in Nigeria, Mali, and Senegal. Over 11,000 EVD victims died in the resulting outbreak in West Africa (WHO data).

A vastly smaller number of patients with EVD received treatment outside of Africa, including 11 in the United States and 16 in Europe.[16] Of these 27 patients, the majority were infected in West Africa, but 2 patients were nurses who were secondarily infected following exposure to a man with EVD who had traveled recently to Liberia. These cases of imported EVD increased awareness of the risk of viral hemorrhagic fe-vers in a globalized world, but, more practically, it also demonstrated to clinicians in industrialized countries the intensity of resources, staffing, and training required to safely care for patients with EVD. The mortality of patients with EVD treated in indus-trialized countries was low compared with the experience in West Africa (5/27 total pa-tients, or 18.5%),[17] with the successful implementation of critical care interventions previously thought to be futile, including mechanical ventilation and renal replacement therapy. At the same time, the low numbers of cases permitted an intensity of care in the United States and Europe that may not be feasible in a generalized outbreak.

Beyond the hospital, Ebola produced a unique public response. Widespread media reporting on the risks of EVD transmission led to public concern and occasional pro-tests,[18] as well as potential stigma and social isolation for international health workers returning home after caring for patients with EVD.[19]

INTENSIVE CARE UNIT PLANNING FOR PANDEMICS

As with any disaster impacting hospitals, the fundamental limitations of "stuff, staff, and space" apply to ICU planning for pandemics. Hospital staff can be and often are impacted personally by noninfectious disasters in their communities, such as hur-ricanes and earthquakes, with effects on their ability to come to work and care for pa-tients.[20,21] In caring for patients with infectious diseases during epidemics, however, much of the risk to HCWs is a direct result of their actual work and not a general risk to their community; as such, training and institutional precautions need to be implemented to both protect staff and reduce absenteeism.[22,23]

"Stuff": Supply Requirements for Pandemic Preparedness

In an epidemic or pandemic, supplies are at increased risk for being depleted rapidly. Per Joint Commission requirements, accredited hospitals in the United States are required to plan for 96 hours of autonomous function without resupply, although this does not imply "full functional capacity" but rather the ability to care for existing patients and staff. Despite this requirement, shortages of routine supplies well within this 96-hour limit have been described in recent disasters.[24]

Disposable items, such as pharmaceuticals (and particularly antimicrobial drugs), may be rapidly exhausted. ICU-specific reusable devices, most notably mechanical ventilators, may similarly be in limited supply, especially in a respiratory disease outbreak. There are approximately 62,000 full-feature ventilators (20 ventilators per 100,000 residents) in the United States. An influenza pandemic with a 30% attack rate and a high case-fatality rate could lead to a doubling of ventilator demand.[25,26] When additional supplies are not available, alternative methods to provide respiratory support may need to be considered, such as the use of anesthesia ventilators, high-flow nasal cannula oxygenation, and noninvasive positive pressure ventilation for selected patients.[27,28]

In light of a known epidemic or pandemic, local, state, and federal health authorities require coordination to assess known available quantities of available required agents, such as oseltamivir and peramivir for influenza, plus appropriate antimicrobial drugs for secondary bacterial infections. In addition, planning needs to include "general" drugs used in the management of critically ill patients, such as intravenous fluids, agents for rapid-sequence intubation, analgesics and sedatives for intubated patients, vasopressors, venous thromboembolism prophylaxis, and neuromuscular blockade agents for patients with severe hypoxemic respiratory failure.

Given ongoing issues with drug shortages in the United States and elsewhere for commonly used agents, planning must also account for the need to identify alternative agents in the event of significant limitations in supply.[29] It is worth noting that not all alternative agents are equivalent in efficacy to preferred first-line therapies, as illustrated in recent US shortages of norepinephrine,[30] although this may be considered acceptable in a pandemic setting.

Although resupply from outside of an affected geographic area may be practical during a localized epidemic, a major pandemic could easily lead to nationwide shortages of routine agents. The US Department of Health and Human Services maintains the Strategic National Stockpile, which includes a stockpile of emergency pharmaceuticals, intravenous fluids, mechanical ventilators, and investigational agents available for emergency use (eg, brincidofovir for a poxvirus outbreak).[31]

High-containment pathogens, such as Ebola have special supply requirements. Ventilators, laboratory equipment, and other routine medical devices need to be specifically dedicated to patients with EVD.[32] Medical waste production for patients with EVD is exceptionally high, with a single patient's management generating enough waste to fill 8 drums (60 L) in 1 day in the Netherlands.[33] Procedures for autoclaving solid waste and decontaminating liquid waste before disposal in municipal systems are mandatory.[34]

"Staff": Increasing the Safety of Trained Personnel

Preserving a hospital's critical care capability during pandemics depends on trained personnel. When faced with an overwhelming number of ill patients, capacity may be increased by having trained critical care personnel supervise staff experienced in acute care (eg, hospitalists, medical/surgical nurses, general inpatient pharmacists), intervening directly for highly complex patients as well as for emergencies and procedures.[35]

HCWs may themselves fall victim to a pandemic, either in the community or at the bedside.[36] In addition to general principles of surge response described elsewhere in this issue, staff safety needs to be maintained through careful infection prevention practices, the use of personal protective equipment (PPE), and medical countermeasures, such as vaccines or chemoprophylaxis as appropriate.

For seasonal influenza outbreaks, droplet precautions (separate rooms without dedicated negative-pressure systems) have been considered adequate. During the H1N1 pandemic, conventional surgical masks seemed sufficient as PPE for HCWs when compared with N95 respirators, although there may have been an advantage to N95 masks for laboratory staff.[37] HCW compliance with influenza vaccination has been historically inadequate; strong encouragement from institutional leadership and consideration for mandatory vaccination may be recommended.[38]

Novel respiratory viruses, such as a novel SARS-like or MERS-like coronavirus, will require novel preventive strategies to maintain staff safety. It is prudent to place such patients into negative-pressure rooms with airborne and contact isolation, with staff wearing N95 respirators, gowns, gloves, and shoe covers until further guidance from national and international public health authorities can be obtained. Active surveillance of patients admitted with respiratory disease, relocation of emergency department triage to a unit outside of the physical hospital, and establishment of dedicated units for patients with confirmed disease are similarly advisable, as was done with the SARS epidemic.[10] Aerosolizing procedures, such as endotracheal intubation, bronchoscopy, and tracheostomy, can be performed using purified air-powered respirators (PAPRs).[10] PAPRs may also be an alternative to N95 masks when negative-pressure isolation rooms are not available in sufficient numbers for affected patients, although formal training in the proper use of these devices is necessary in advance.

Ebola and other high-containment pathogens require higher levels of expertise and precaution than even a respiratory virus. Following intensive initial training, the care of patients with EVD requires regular refresher training, with dedicated space for patient and staff safety as well as waste management, laboratory diagnostics, and the like. Full contact precautions and the use of PAPRs are routine in most US Ebola treatment units (ETUs). Training for hospital staff is available through the National Ebola Training and Education Center (www.netec.org).

Although having an adequate number of trained personnel is critical during an epidemic, "presenteeism," the act of coming to work while ill, is a significant threat to staff safety. Surveys during previous influenza years reported that over 40% of HCWs might come to work while suffering from respiratory infections, increasing the risk of transmission to staff and to patients.[39] Even in settings of potential staff shortages, institutions must maintain policies to prevent HCWs with symptoms of the disease to avoid work and to seek appropriate medical care for themselves.

"Space": Critical Care Without an Intensive Care Unit

Although the practice of critical care is generally linked to the ICU as a location, critically ill patients may need to receive care outside of a traditional ICU in disaster settings. Considerations of infection prevention and the avoidance of cross-contamination may additionally dictate that infected patients be placed in a geographically separate location. In situations where there are inadequate numbers of individual

---

Box 1
Planning for pandemics

1. Triage and resource allocation. If a disease outbreak overwhelms local capacity, even at surge levels, institutions will need to determine a just allocation of scarce resources. If hospital transfer outside of the affected region is possible, this will require coordination by regional and national authorities. Scarce resources, such as ECMO or access to an ETU, will require allocation in a manner that is open, consistent, and based on broadly accepted ethical principles. These decisions will benefit from intensivist input but cannot be the sole decision of intensivists. Critical care admission may need to be limited to patients with reasonable chances of survival, along with the use of ventilators if in shortage. The states of New York[43] and Maryland[44] have published ventilator allocation guidelines that use community engagement to best reflect local priorities and values. In all cases, critically ill patients denied ICU admission in a disaster must receive appropriate and compassionate palliative care.

2. Optimization of staffing. For hospitals that maintain an ETU capability, regular refresher training must be exercised to preserve perishable skills. For all hospitals, appropriate staff training on infection prevention practices for pandemic threats are a key part of training; "just-in-time" training in the event of an outbreak may be needed to augment routine training, but a core group of staff trained in pandemic diseases, including donning and doffing of PPE and PAPR use, should be routine for institutions.

3. Equipment, supplies, and space. In addition to maintaining the Joint Commission-mandated 96-hour supply requirement (including food, water, consumables, and medications), hospitals should have plans for obtaining additional supplies in coordination with nearby hospitals, pharmaceutical vendors, and regional and national health authorities, including via the Strategic National Stockpile. PAPRs, negative-pressure rooms, and anticipated bed capacity in different surge levels should be defined in advance. These surge plans need to include plans for alternate care sites within the institution for ICU-level patients, such as PACUs, as noted above, as well as plans for transfer for patients when capabilities are ultimately overwhelmed. Lastly, hospitals must ensure proper staff vaccination and discourage "presenteeism" for ill personnel.

4. Public health. Hospitals and ICUs must have plans to coordinate with public health authorities for identification of cases, access to diagnostics, and tracking of potentially contagious individuals as part of outbreak investigations. Systematic data collection, either through government, academic, or combined networks, is similarly crucial to test interventions to end an epidemic.

5. Public affairs. Hospitals should be transparent in their interactions with communities, while also protecting the privacy and dignity of their patients. In addition to community involvement in ethical decision-making, such as ventilator allocation, media interactions need to be done with the oversight of hospital administration, experienced public affairs personnel, and ideally in collaboration with public health authorities.

---

rooms, patients with confirmed infections may be cohorted in common areas to reduce the risk of cross-contamination.[40]

During a standard hospital surge, it is anticipated that institutions can tolerate a 20% increase in critically ill patients with minimal impact. Increases of up to 200% of normal capacity may occur, but only at the cost of degraded capability and a possible modification in the standard of care. When ICU capacity is exceeded, less-ill patients may need to be transferred to other levels of care, such as patients not requiring mechanical ventilation, vasopressor support, or intensive neuromonitoring. Conversely, areas of the hospital capable of ICU-level monitoring, such as a postanesthesia care unit (PACU) or a monitored step-down unit, may need to be repurposed as temporary ICUs, especially if cohorting of seriously ill patients is planned. (Cancellation of elective surgical procedures may open up the PACU and same-day surgical units as auxiliary ICUs and step-down units, for example.)

Ebola and other high-containment pathogens require even-more specific dedicated space. As of 2016, there were 56 Centers for Disease Control and Prevention-designated ETUs in the United States, not of all which have maintained their capabilities since the end of the West Africa epidemic.[41] Space (and staff) allocation for the care of a single patient with EVD in a US ETU may require the loss of 6 or more "standard" beds in terms of capacity.[41] Because the total number of designated ETU beds in the United States is less than 100, it would take relatively few patients with EVD or similarly contagious diseases to rapidly overwhelm current national capacity.[42]

PLANNING FOR PANDEMICS

The appropriate response to epidemics and pandemics, like any disaster, requires appropriate planning by ICUs and their associated hospitals. The precise response will necessarily vary based on the scale and severity of the pandemic (**Box 1**).

SUMMARY

Pandemics and epidemics are unique challenges for ICU preparedness. In a highly mobile, globalized world, infectious disease is no longer confined to fixed geographic regions. The risks of pandemic disease to clinical staff requires that institutions have mechanisms to protect their personnel while also providing adequate care to affected patients. Engagement of community partners is necessary to permit adequate data collection, to develop ethical standards for resource allocation, and to manage anxiety and expectations among the public.

REFERENCES

1. Hung LS. The SARS epidemic in Hong Kong: what lessons have we learned? J R Soc Med 2003;96:374–8.
2. Wong ATY, Chen H, Liu SH, et al. From SARS to avian influenza preparedness in Hong Kong. Clin Infect Dis 2017;64:S98–104.
3. Christian MD, Poutanen SM, Loutfy MR, et al. Severe acute respiratory syndrome. Clin Infect Dis 2004;38:1420–7.
4. Centers for Disease Control and Prevention. Update: outbreak of severe acute respiratory syndrome–worldwide, 2003. MMWR Morb Mortal Wkly Rep 2003;52:241–6, 8.
5. Varia M, Wilson S, Sarwal S, et al. Investigation of a nosocomial outbreak of severe acute respiratory syndrome (SARS) in Toronto, Canada. CMAJ 2003;169:285–92.
6. Lew TW, Kwek TK, Tai D, et al. Acute respiratory distress syndrome in critically ill patients with severe acute respiratory syndrome. JAMA 2003;290:374–80.
7. Booth CM, Matukas LM, Tomlinson GA, et al. Clinical features and short-term outcomes of 144 patients with SARS in the greater Toronto area. JAMA 2003;289:2801–9.
8. Centers for Disease Control and Prevention (CDC). Severe acute respiratory syndrome (SARS) and coronavirus testing–United States, 2003. MMWR Morb Mortal Wkly Rep 2003;52:297–302.
9. Tsang KW, Ho PL, Ooi GC, et al. A cluster of cases of severe acute respiratory syndrome in Hong Kong. N Engl J Med 2003;348:1977–85.

10. Cheng VC, Chan JF, To KK, et al. Clinical management and infection control of SARS: lessons learned. Antiviral Res 2013;100:407–19.
11. Ofner-Agostini M, Wallington T, Henry B, et al. Investigation of the second wave (phase 2) of severe acute respiratory syndrome (SARS) in Toronto, Canada. What happened? Can Commun Dis Rep 2008;34:1–11.
12. Dominguez-Cherit G, Lapinsky SE, Macias AE, et al. Critically ill patients with 2009 influenza A(H1N1) in Mexico. JAMA 2009;302:1880–7.
13. Dawood FS, Iuliano AD, Reed C, et al. Estimated global mortality associated with the first 12 months of 2009 pandemic influenza A H1N1 virus circulation: a modelling study. Lancet Infect Dis 2012;12:687–95.
14. Investigators AI, Webb SA, Pettila V, et al. Critical care services and 2009 H1N1 influenza in Australia and New Zealand. N Engl J Med 2009;361:1925–34.
15. Kumar A, Zarychanski R, Pinto R, et al. Critically ill patients with 2009 influenza A(H1N1) infection in Canada. JAMA 2009;302:1872–9.
16. Leligdowicz A, Fischer WA 2nd, Uyeki TM, et al. Ebola virus disease and critical illness. Crit Care 2016;20:217.
17. Uyeki TM, Mehta AK, Davey RT Jr, et al. Clinical management of Ebola virus disease in the United States and Europe. N Engl J Med 2016;374:636–46.
18. Sell TK, Boddie C, McGinty EE, et al. Media messages and perception of risk for Ebola virus infection, United States. Emerg Infect Dis 2017;23:108–11.
19. Gee S, Skovdal M. Public discourses of Ebola contagion and courtesy stigma: the real risk to international health care workers returning home from the West Africa Ebola outbreak? Qual Health Res 2018;28:1499–508.
20. Morris AM, Ricci KA, Griffin AR, et al. Personal and professional challenges confronted by hospital staff following hurricane sandy: a qualitative assessment of management perspectives. BMC Emerg Med 2016;16:18.
21. Ochi S, Tsubokura M, Kato S, et al. Hospital staff shortage after the 2011 triple disaster in Fukushima, Japan - an earthquake, tsunamis, and nuclear power plant accident: a case of the Soso district. PLoS One 2016;11:e0164952.
22. Shiao JS, Koh D, Lo LH, et al. Factors predicting nurses' consideration of leaving their job during the SARS outbreak. Nurs Ethics 2007;14:5–17.
23. Maunder RG, Lancee WJ, Balderson KE, et al. Long-term psychological and occupational effects of providing hospital healthcare during SARS outbreak. Emerg Infect Dis 2006;12:1924–32.
24. Abramson DM, Redlener I. Hurricane sandy: lessons learned, again. Disaster Med Public Health Prep 2012;6:328–9.
25. Meltzer MI, Patel A, Ajao A, et al. Estimates of the demand for mechanical ventilation in the United States during an influenza pandemic. Clin Infect Dis 2015;60(Suppl 1):S52–7.
26. Rubinson L, Vaughn F, Nelson S, et al. Mechanical ventilators in US acute care hospitals. Disaster Med Public Health Prep 2010;4:199–206.
27. Rubinson L, Branson RD, Pesik N, et al. Positive-pressure ventilation equipment for mass casualty respiratory failure. Biosecur Bioterror 2006;4:183–94.
28. Papazian L, Corley A, Hess D, et al. Use of high-flow nasal cannula oxygenation in ICU adults: a narrative review. Intensive Care Med 2016;42:1336–49.
29. Mazer-Amirshahi M, Goyal M, Umar SA, et al. U.S. drug shortages for medications used in adult critical care (2001-2016). J Crit Care 2017;41:283–8.
30. Vail E, Gershengorn HB, Hua M, et al. Association between US norepinephrine shortage and mortality among patients with septic shock. JAMA 2017;317:1433–42.

31. Redd SC, Frieden TR. CDC's evolving approach to emergency response. Health Secur 2017;15:41–52.
32. Garibaldi BT, Chertow DS. High-containment pathogen preparation in the intensive care unit. Infect Dis Clin North Am 2017;31:561–76.
33. Haverkort JJ, Minderhoud AL, Wind JD, et al. Hospital preparations for viral hemorrhagic fever patients and experience gained from admission of an Ebola patient. Emerg Infect Dis 2016;22:184–91.
34. Le AB, Hoboy S, Germain A, et al. A pilot survey of the U.S. medical waste industry to determine training needs for safely handling highly infectious waste. Am J Infect Control 2018;46:133–8.
35. Einav S, Hick JL, Hanfling D, et al. Surge capacity logistics: care of the critically ill and injured during pandemics and disasters: CHEST consensus statement. Chest 2014;146:e17S–43S.
36. Suwantarat N, Apisarnthanarak A. Risks to healthcare workers with emerging diseases: lessons from MERS-CoV, Ebola, SARS, and avian flu. Curr Opin Infect Dis 2015;28:349–61.
37. Smith JD, MacDougall CC, Johnstone J, et al. Effectiveness of N95 respirators versus surgical masks in protecting health care workers from acute respiratory infection: a systematic review and meta-analysis. CMAJ 2016;188:567–74.
38. Bellia C, Setbon M, Zylberman P, et al. Healthcare worker compliance with seasonal and pandemic influenza vaccination. Influenza Other Respir Viruses 2013;7(Suppl 2):97–104.
39. Chiu S, Black CL, Yue X, et al. Working with influenza-like illness: presenteeism among US health care personnel during the 2014-2015 influenza season. Am J Infect Control 2017;45:1254–8.
40. Prevention strategies for seasonal influenza in healthcare settings. Available at: https://www.cdc.gov/flu/professionals/infectioncontrol/healthcaresettings.htm. Accessed March 02, 2019.
41. Herstein JJ, Biddinger PD, Gibbs SG, et al. Sustainability of high-level isolation capabilities among US Ebola treatment centers. Emerg Infect Dis 2017;23:965–7.
42. Herstein JJ, Biddinger PD, Kraft CS, et al. Current capabilities and capacity of Ebola treatment centers in the United States. Infect Control Hosp Epidemiol 2016;37:313–8.
43. Powell T, Christ KC, Birkhead GS. Allocation of ventilators in a public health disaster. Disaster Med Public Health Prep 2008;2:20–6.
44. Daugherty Biddison EL, Faden R, Gwon HS, et al. Too many patients...A framework to guide statewide allocation of scarce mechanical ventilation during disasters. Chest 2019;155(4):848–54.

Disasters Resulting from Radiologic and Nuclear Events

John S. Parrish, MD*, Gilbert Seda, MD, PhD

KEYWORDS

- Acute radiation syndrome • Radiation injury • Biodosimetry • Internal contamination
- Chelating agents • Colony-stimulating factors

KEY POINTS

- Radiation accidents and incidents although rare have the potential to produce large numbers of casualties with predictable patterns of injury.
- After stabilization of life-threatening injuries, patients should undergo external decontamination before entry into the health care facility.
- An accurate estimate of whole-body exposure received by an individual can be obtained from an assessment of the time to onset of prodromal symptoms, the rate of depletion of lymphocytes, and the results of a lymphocyte dicentric assay.
- Acute radiation syndrome may manifest as 3 unique subsyndromes representing damage to the hematopoietic, gastrointestinal, and central nervous systems.
- Patients who have received 4 to 8 Gy of whole-body radiation can be expected to benefit from ICU-based aggressive treatment. Patients who receive more than 10 to 12 Gy of whole-body irradiation are unlikely to survive even when aggressive treatment is provided.
- The management of acute radiation syndrome is mainly supportive, and includes fluids, antibiotics, blood products, and, in certain cases, colony-stimulating factors and stem cell transplant.

INTRODUCTION

Accidents or terrorist incidents involving ionizing radiation have the potential to produce large numbers of casualties. Since 1945, more than 500 major radiation accidents have been reported worldwide. These events have occurred due to laboratory accidents, industrial accidents, accidents during transportation of radioactive material, improper disposal of material, accidents during medical use, and power plant

Disclosure: The authors have nothing to disclose.
Department of Pulmonary and Critical Care Medicine, Naval Medical Center San Diego, 34800 Bob Wilson Drive, Suite 301, San Diego, CA 92134, USA
* Corresponding author.
E-mail address: jscottpccm@gmail.com

Crit Care Clin 35 (2019) 619–631
https://doi.org/10.1016/j.ccc.2019.06.005
0749-0704/19/Published by Elsevier Inc.
criticalcare.theclinics.com

mishaps.[1] These accidents have typically produced small numbers of casualties. The 1986 Chernobyl nuclear power plant accident, causing a huge release of radionuclides over large areas of Belarus, Ukraine, and the Russian Federation, was the most severe in the history of the nuclear power industry. As a result of this event, more than 130 patients developed the acute radiation syndrome.[2] Since 9/11 the potential for terrorist events involving radioactive material has mandated that these possibilities be incorporated into emergency management planning. Possible terrorist events that should be considered include the use of a radioactive exposure device (RED); the detonation of a radiologic dispersal device (RDD/dirty bomb); an attack on a nuclear power plant; the detonation of an improvised nuclear device; or the detonation of a nuclear weapon. REDs are radioactive materials that are covertly placed with the intention of exposing victims to harmful radiation. The potential dangers of the deployment of a RED depends on the type and amount of radioactive material present, the duration of exposure, and the proximity of the source to the victims. Unexplained burns, cytopenias, or unexplained nausea and vomiting should alert clinicians to the possible presence of a RED. Combining radioactive material with conventional explosives is used to construct an RDD/dirty bomb. Sources for this device could be potentially obtained from medical facilities, laboratories, industry, or improperly stored nuclear wastes. Given the expected amount of radioactive material used in a dirty bomb, it is anticipated that the use of this sort of device will produce most casualties from traditional blast injuries, with acute radiation effects being less likely. An exception to this would be victims who present with imbedded radioactive fragments. These fragments can be highly radioactive and can rapidly cause significant radionecrosis of surrounding tissue if not removed promptly. The successful detonation of an RDD would be expected to cause significant social and psychologic injuries to the affected population. The detonation of a nuclear device results from nuclear fission or thermonuclear fusion, during this process a tremendous amount of energy is released in the form of blast, heat, and radiation. This energy release would subject the affected population to life-threatening radiation exposures, thermal burns, and blast injuries.[3–5]

BASIC RADIATION PHYSICS

Radiation is defined as energy that is transmitted through space in the form of high-speed particles or electromagnetic waves. This energy can be ionizing or nonionizing. Ionizing radiation is any electromagnetic or particulate radiation capable of producing ions, either directly or indirectly, by interaction with matter. Nonionizing radiation does not create ions or charged particles. Ionizing radiation is more harmful to humans than nonionizing radiation, and is the type of radiation that is of concern in a radiologic or nuclear event. The 4 most common forms of ionizing radiation are: alpha, beta, gamma, and neutrons. Alpha particles are positively charged, have mass, and are blocked by thin barriers such as paper, clothing, and skin. Alpha particles do not typically represent an external hazard but, when ingested, they have the potential to cause significant organ damage. Beta particles are negatively charged electrons that can travel short distances in tissue. They are typically blocked by wood or concrete. They can result in external hazards after prolonged exposure. Beta particles are also harmful when ingested or inhaled. Gamma rays are electromagnetic, have no mass, and readily penetrate tissue. They present significant external hazards depending on the duration of exposure, distance from the source, and presence or absence of shielding. Neutrons, such as gamma rays, are uncharged. They are typically produced only by nuclear reactors or nuclear detonations. They can penetrate tissues deeply and represent an extreme external hazard. Ionizing radiation interacts with the human body via direct and indirect mechanisms. Radiation has the potential to directly damage critical biological molecules, and indirectly affects tissue by producing ions and free radicals that then interact with cellular components.

The absorbed dose of ionizing radiation is traditionally measured in rad (radiation absorbed dose). The international unit Gray (Gy) is equivalent to 100 rad. Owing to varying biological effects of the different types of ionizing radiation, the dose-equivalent unit rem (roentgen equivalent man), international unit Sievert, is used for assessing radiation damage to tissues. Depending on the nature of the event radiation injury can occur from external irradiation, external contamination with radioactive materials, internal contamination, or any combination of these. A patient who has only been irradiated is not radioactive and does not pose a risk to others. Contaminated patients have radioisotopes on or in the body and are radioactive, therefore they present an ongoing exposure risk to themselves as well as others.[6,7]

PATTERNS OF INJURY FROM RADIATION

The types and severity of injuries caused by a radiologic event depend on several factors, such as the total dose received, the rate at which it is delivered, the type of radiation (alpha, beta, gamma, or neutrons) and the radiosensitivity and volume of tissue irradiated. Health effects resulting from radiation are of 2 general types, stochastic and deterministic. The stochastic effect of primary concern is carcinogenesis. Deterministic or nonstochastic effects in an organ, by contrast, arise from radiation-induced damage to susceptible cells. Tissues with rapidly dividing cells or with high metabolic activity are commonly more sensitive to radiation-induced cell killing and resultant deterministic effects. Nonproliferating or slowly proliferating cells, such as those of the liver, kidneys, blood vessels, and connective tissues are less radiosensitive to cell killing. Organ dysfunction is seen when ionizing radiation disables or kills so many of its essential or proliferative cells that it ceases to function properly. Such an effect will be seen with a reasonable degree of certainty if a dose that exceeds an organ-specific threshold dose is delivered over a short period of time. Once the threshold is exceeded the severity of the response in the tissue grows exponentially with dose. Acute effects can be apparent within minutes to hours to days depending on the dose received. A uniform whole-body dose of 0.3 Gy from an external exposure of penetrating radiation delivered over a matter of minutes is likely to cause only mild symptoms, specifically nausea and perhaps vomiting. At higher doses significant organ dysfunction can be seen. Whole-body doses of 3.5 to 4 Gy will result in death in 50% of the victims when supportive therapy is not available. With treatment, the median lethal dose increases from 6 to 7 Gy. When compared with whole-body exposures, equivalent doses of radiation delivered to isolated portions of the body, that is, extremities, would not be expected to have such high mortality owing to the preservation of significant portions of the bone marrow.

The acute radiation syndrome (ARS) is a broad term used to describe a range of signs and symptoms that reflect severe damage to specific organ systems and that can lead to death within hours to months after exposure. Three distinct clusters of symptoms arising from damage to 3 separate biologic compartments point to the onset of ARS. These subsyndromes are known as the hematopoietic syndrome, the gastrointestinal syndrome, and the central nervous system or cardiovascular syndrome, and they are seen with increasing whole-body dose in this respective order. The hematopoietic subsyndrome occurs following acute radiation exposures greater than 1 Gy. At higher doses symptoms will overlap for each of the acute subsyndromes.

Disease progression over time has classically been divided into 4 stages: prodromal, latent, manifest illness, and recovery or death. These stages are distinct and the timing and severity of clinical effects of each is strongly dependent on the dose received. After a significant dose of radiation, symptoms of ARS usually present early as the pro-dromal stage, also called the "N-V-D" (nausea, vomiting, and diarrhea) stage. These initial signs, which may also include fatigability, headache, anorexia, parotitis, erythema, and fever are similar for all ARS syndromes, but their severity and speed of onset depends on the dose received. This prodromal stage is followed by the symptom-free latent stage, during which the patient may appear and feel relatively well. The duration of the latency stage is inversely proportional to the dose and lasts for 1 to 3 weeks for survivable exposures. Absence of a latent phase is suggestive of a nonsurvivable radiation injury. The latent stage is followed by the manifest illness stage. This stage may appear within days to months after the exposure and the onset is again dependent on the initial dose.

Finally, recovery for a survivor is a function of the initial mechanism of injury and whole-body exposure. Recuperation can take weeks to years. For those who do not recover, death may occur within hours to months and is again is dependent on the dose initially received. The cutaneous syndrome may occur in isolation or may be present with other symptoms if there is significant widespread or local irradiation of the skin. Symptoms and signs of the cutaneous syndrome typically appear several days after the exposure. Multiple organ dysfunction syndrome, defined as progressive dysfunction of 2 or more organs over time, has been described in association with acute radiation exposures. Late deterministic effects, such as fibrosis and cataracts can occur. Due to immunosuppression and delayed tissue healing associated with significant radiation exposures, patients with coexistent trauma or burns will have a significantly worse prognosis.[7,8]

INITIAL ASSESSMENT AND MANAGEMENT

Initial medical care for all casualties of a radiologic event will include resuscitation and treatment of life-threatening injuries, triage, and decontamination. The treatment of acute life-threatening injuries has priority over decontamination and the management of the radiation-associated injuries.[9] After initial stabilization, patients will undergo initial external decontamination at the scene. **Fig. 1**, provides a standard outline for the initial management of casualties from a radiation event.

DECONTAMINATION

Radiation casualties should be promptly decontaminated to decrease additional radiation exposure to the victims, and to prevent contamination of other patients, medical personnel, and the health care facility. Following stabilization of life-threatening injuries, decontamination should occur in a specially designated area that is outside the hospital. This area should be situated downwind of the treatment facility.

All health care workers should protect themselves with scrubs, gowns, masks, double gloves, and shoe covers during the treatment and decontamination of radiation casualties. The outer gloves should be changed frequently to minimize cross-contamination. These standard measures provide sufficient protection from any radio-active isotopes that could be contaminating a patient. It is best to assume that every patient near a radiation exposure event is contaminated until proven otherwise.

The decontamination process is straightforward. All of the patient's clothing is removed and discarded into a clearly labeled and secure container so that it does not contaminate other people and the surroundings. If the clothing needs to be cut

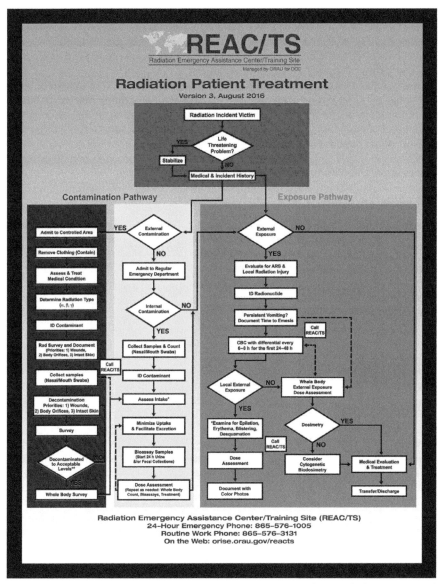

Fig. 1. REAC/TS patient treatment algorithm. [a] See REAC/TS Pocket Guide http://orise.oral. gov/reacts/resources/radiation-accident-management-aspx. [b] <2-3X Natural Background or No Reduction in Counts, Medical Priorities Dictato Stopping Decontamination, Health Physics Consultation Warranted. (*Courtesy of* Oak Ridge Institute for Science and Education.)

off the patient, the scissors should be washed with soap and water frequently to avoid spreading contamination. After all clothing has been removed; the patient is thoroughly washed with soap and water. The removal of all clothing followed by a simple soap and water wash is effective in removing more than 95% of residual radioactive material from externally contaminated patients. Patients would then undergo whole-body radiation survey with radiologic survey instruments. If areas of external contamination persist, then the soap and water wash should be repeated. After whole-body decontamination of the skin, then radioactive shrapnel, open wounds, and body entrance cavities should be decontaminated. Areas of residual external radiation should be covered with waterproof dressings to limit spread of contamination to other body sites, the environment, and other personnel.

Once a radiation-exposed patient has been stabilized and decontaminated, he or she should be triaged, and admitted to the hospital when appropriate for definitive care. It is recommended that all radiation casualties be admitted to specially designated areas of the hospital and that the staff in these areas wear appropriate protective clothing as described previously.

Patients who have ingested, inhaled, or absorbed radioisotopes should undergo initial treatment for internal contamination as soon as possible.[7,10,11]

DOSE ESTIMATION/TRIAGE

An early accurate whole-body dose estimate is crucial to the triage of patients with acute radiation exposures during a disaster. This dose estimate allows optimal use of limited resources. Three main elements that are essential for estimating the dose are vomiting onset time, kinetics of depletion of lymphocytes, and chromosome abnormalities. Cytogenetic biodosimetry is considered the "gold standard" for determination of whole-body dose, but no single assay is accurate enough to address all potential radiation scenarios. Given the limitations of individual assays, it is recommended that multiple parameters (symptoms, lymphocyte depletion kinetics, and biodosimetry/cytogenetics) be used to guide triage. There are several online triage tools available to assist with dose estimates.[12–14] When available, other tests such as electron paramagnetic resonance of teeth, nails, and hair, when available, can be extremely helpful in the accurate assessment of whole-body dose estimations.[15] It is important to remember that it is the whole-body dose that is most crucial to accurately predict prognosis. Relatively large radiation doses delivered to extremities are potentially survivable if significant portions of the bone marrow are spared.

Early onset emesis, as well as a rapid decrease in lymphocyte count, is consistent with a lethal dose. Survival is highly likely for patients who have received less than 1 Gy of radiation and have minimal associated injuries. These patients may be managed as outpatients or in a ward setting. Patients who have received 2 to 8 Gy may benefit from the aggressive treatment available in an intensive care unit (ICU). In a limited casualty situation, patients with exposures who have significant cutaneous, gastrointestinal, and neurovascular symptoms should be triaged to the ICU. Patients who have received moderate doses of radiation and develop multiorgan failure days to weeks after the event may benefit from ICU care. Patients whose estimated whole-body doses are greater than 10 to 12 Gy should receive comfort measures, because more aggressive care will not affect outcomes for this group of patients who have received a lethal dose of radiation. **Table 1** provides useful guidance to assist with the triage of casualties.[16–20]

MANAGEMENT OF INTERNAL CONTAMINATION

Internal contamination, which can result from the inhalation, ingestion, injection, or transdermal penetration of radioactive material, is the presence of radioisotopes within the body. It is an ongoing exposure risk to the patient. Internal organs commonly affected by internal radiation contamination are the thyroid, the lung, the liver, adipose tissue, and bone.

Table 1
Radiologic triage considerations

Triage Category	Unaffected <0.75 Gy	Minimal 0.75–2 Gy	Variable 2–3 Gy	Urgent 3–6 Gy	Immediate 6–10 Gy[a]	Expectant >10 Gy[a]
Symptomatology	Unlikely to cause any acute symptoms	May lead to mild and delayed symptoms	Likely to lead to moderate to severe symptoms	Likely to lead to early severe symptoms with potential for lethal outcome	Likely to lead to early excruciating symptoms and mortality without substantial treatment	Likely to lead to early death
Appropriate care setting	CBTF	CBTF, outpatient medical care follow-up	Outpatient medical care, possible inpatient	Inpatient, possible ICU	Extended ICU critical care	ICU
ARS subsyndrome	Unlikely	Mild hematopoietic	Hematopoietic	Severe hematopoietic and mild gastrointestinal	Severe hematopoietic and severe gastrointestinal	Severe hematopoietic and severe gastrointestinal and onset of cerebrovascular
Medical management	Counseling	Counseling, provide dose-response symptom information	Antibiotics	Extended antibiotics, cytokines and AED	Extended antibiotics, cytokines, AED. antidiarrheals, anti-emetics, oral and IV nutrition, fluids, universal precautions, consider SCT	Balance fluid management with gastrointestinal and cerebrovascular symptoms, SCT, likely palliative care
Clinical resource burden, impact	Minimal, CBTF designed to address population needs	Low, outpatient care and public health stressed	Moderate, outpatient care stressed	Moderate, inpatient care stressed	Highly clinical resource intensive, ICU and extended stress on inpatient resources	Extremely clinical resource intensive, extensive stress on ICU assets

Abbreviations: AED, adrenocortical steroid hormone to stimulate immune response; CBTF, community-based treatment facility; SCT, hematopoietic-stem cell transplantation.

[a] Recommend immediate care triage category modified to 8 Gy in mass casualty scenario when clinical resources are limited (eg, immediate care exposure dose range 6–8 Gy and expectant >8 Gy).

From Rea M, Gougelet R, Nicolalde R, Geiling J, Swartz H. Proposed triage categories for large-scale radiation incidents using high-accuracy biodosimetry methods. Health Physics. 2010;98(2):136-144.

INITIAL ASSESSMENT FOR INTERNAL CONTAMINATION

Patients who have inhaled or ingested material, have significant external contamination, or have open wounds should be evaluated for possible internal contamination. The specific isotopes involved in the radiation incident should be identified. An initial survey of the patient with a radiac meter should be performed with attention to the mouth, nose, and wounds. Radioactive material found on nasal and oral swabs will help to identify patients with internal contamination. The collection of stool and urine samples can be very helpful in determining both the type and the amount of internal radiation that an individual might have received. Bronchoalveolar lavage samples can be obtained when indicated. Whole-body radiation surveys can be used to determine the extent of any internal radiation contamination. The analysis of nasal swabs, stool samples, and urine samples are the most practical methods of determining the type and extent of internal radiation contamination by hospital-based physicians.

TREATMENT OF INTERNAL RADIATION CONTAMINATION

Patients with internal radiation contamination should be promptly treated to reduce the absorbed radiation dose. The goals of treatment are to reduce absorption and enhance elimination of the internal radionuclide contaminant. There are 3 main categories of agents that are used to treat internal radiation contamination: purgative agents, blocking agents, and chelation agents. Specific radiation countermeasures for treatment of internal contamination are dependent on the specific radioactive isotopes present. Treatment is most effective when given as early as possible after exposure. Gastric lavage preformed early can be used to empty the stomach after the potential ingestion of radionuclides. If promptly performed, gastric lavage should decrease the concentration of radionuclides in the gastrointestinal tract. Bronchoalveolar lavage has been shown to be effective in removing inhaled radioactive isotopes from the lungs of animals and should be considered when significant internal contamination of the lungs is suspected. Purgative agents are used to remove radionuclides from the gastrointestinal tract. The most common purgatives are laxatives and enemas, which are helpful in reducing the transit time of radionuclides in the colon. Agents can be used to bind radioisotopes in the gastrointestinal tract to prevent their uptake. For example, Prussian blue (ferric ferrocyanide) is an ion exchange resin that binds ^{137}cesium in the gastrointestinal tract and facilitates its secretion. Patients who have experienced internal ^{137}cesium should be treated with oral Prussian blue (3 g, 3 times daily). Aluminum hydroxide can be used to bind ^{90}strontium in the gastrointestinal tract. A single 100-mL oral dose of aluminum phosphate gel will block intestinal absorption of ^{90}strontium.

The most important blocking agent is potassium iodide, which is used for $^{125/131}$iodine exposures. Potassium iodide blocks the uptake of radioactive iodine by increasing the uptake of the nonradioactive isotope. Because the thyroid gland is very sensitive to the effects of internal contamination with $^{125/131}$iodine, potassium iodide should be given as soon as possible after radioactive iodine exposure. The recommended dose and duration depend on the projected thyroid dose. Potassium iodide can be taken prophylactically if there is sufficient warning of a potential $^{125/131}$iodine exposure. The standard adult prophylactic dose is a single 130-mg dose of potassium.

Several chelation agents have been used in the treatment of patients with internal contamination. A complete review is beyond the scope of this article. Chelation agents are substances that bind strongly with certain isotopes to form a stable, soluble complex that can be excreted by the kidneys. Diethylenetriaminepentaacetic acid (DTPA) is the most effective and commonly recommended chelation agent for the treatment of internal radiation contamination. DTPA chelation therapy is effective for the treatment of internal radiation contamination with americium, californium, cobalt, curium, pluto-nium, and yttrium. DTPA is administered as a slow IV push of an intravenous solution of 1 g dissolved in 5 mL 5% dextrose in water or 1 g in 250 mL of saline or D5W, infused over 30 minutes. The duration of therapy depends on total body burden and response to treatment. DTPA can be given via nebulized inhalation for treatment of in-ternal contamination of the respiratory tract. Internal contamination with ^{235}uranium can be treated with oral or IV sodium bicarbonate, with the dose regulated to maintain an alkaline urine pH. Excretion of $^{238-235}$uranium can be further enhanced with the addition of a diuretic, such as furosemide. Dimercaprol is a chelation agent that has been used to treat internal contamination with ^{210}polonium.[5] For specific recommen-dations, current treatment guidelines should be consulted.[21-23]

HOSPITAL AND CRITICAL CARE MANAGEMENT

Following resuscitation, stabilization of life-threatening injuries, triage, and initial decontamination, patients with significant acute radiation exposures will be admitted for further management. Standard supportive care includes fluids and electrolyte replacement; antiemetic agents to manage vomiting; antidiarrheal agents to manage diarrhea; proton pump inhibitors for gastrointestinal ulcer prophylaxis; and pain man-agement. Care should be taken to prevent the development of infection or bleeding by avoiding unnecessary instrumentations particularly involving the gastrointestinal tract and the skin.

The clinical management of patients with treatable ARS is primarily based on providing advanced supportive care, while awaiting the affected organ to recover. A main objective is to avoid neutropenia, which can lead to sepsis. Patients with severe bone marrow damage will require fluids, blood products, strict infection control measures, reverse isolation, appropriate prophylactic and advanced antimicrobial therapy, colony-stimulating factors (CSFs), and possible allogenic stem cell transplantation. Bone marrow or stem cell transplantation may have a role in a select group of patients. Blood products should be irradiated and leukoreduced to prevent posttransfusion graft versus host disease. Epoetin and darbepoetin should be considered for patients with anemia.

Hematopoietic growth factors or CSFs are endogenous glycoproteins that stimulate the bone marrow stem cells to mature into blood cell types. The basis for the use of CSFs in patients exposed to radiation is derived from studies followed in patients with cancer, in that small cohort of radiation-exposed victims, and in several prospec-tive trials in canines and nonhuman primates exposed to radiation. The goals of ther-apy are to shorten the duration of severe neutropenia and minimize the severity of neutropenia-associated complications. The cytokine therapies should be strongly considered for children and patients with significant comorbidities who have received greater than 2 Gy whole-body exposure, or significant partial body exposures, and are likely to have an absolute neutrophil count of 500 cells/mm^3 or less. All patients who have documented whole-body exposures greater than 3 Gy should receive cytokine therapy. CSFs should be administered prophylactically as soon as possible after sus-pected or confirmed exposure to radiation doses greater than 2 Gy. The CSF can be discontinued when the neutrophil reaches a level greater than 1000 cells/mL after re-covery from the nadir. Various types of granulocyte colony-CSF (G-CSF) can be given: G-CSF (Filgrastim), pegylated G-CSF (Pegfilgrastim), or GM-CSF (Sargramostim). These are all commercially available preparations and used in the management of hematopoietic subsyndromes.[24-26]

The role of antibiotics in the management of ARS depends on the patient's absorbed radiation dose, absolute neutrophil counts, and potential sources of infection. Susceptibility to infection arises from breeches in the integument or mucosal barriers as well as the presence of neutropenia. In nonneutropenic patients, antibiotics should be directed toward known foci of infection. Prophylactic antibiotics to include antifungals and antivirals should be considered for patients with radiation-induced neutropenia.[27] Infectious Diseases Society of America guidelines should be consulted for use of antibiotics in febrile neutropenic patients.[28]

Blood transfusions are indicated for patients with an acute radiation subsyndrome who have severe bone marrow damage or who require concurrent trauma resuscitation. In the absence of trauma, blood transfusions are not typically required until 2 to 4 weeks after exposure. All cellular products in the blood to be transfused should be leukoreduced and irradiated to 25 Gy to prevent the development of transfusion-related graft versus host disease.

Stem cell transplantation should be considered for certain patients with acute radiation illness if marrow recovery is considered unlikely.[29-32]

MANAGEMENT ISSUES OF THE PATIENT WITH RADIATION INJURY AND TRAUMA

The management of patients with combined acute radiation and trauma present many unique challenges. Because of immunosuppression and delayed tissue healing associated with significant radiation exposures, patients with coexistent trauma or burns will have a significantly worse prognosis. This worsening of prognosis will result in many patients who have severe trauma and significant acute radiation exposures to be triaged to expectant categories. In patients who are deemed to have potentially survivable injuries, the goal of surgery is to complete all procedures within the first 48 hours and to choose techniques that minimize skin entry points. If surgery is not performed in this "window of opportunity" following acute radiation exposure, it may have to be postponed for up to 2 to 3 months until full hematopoietic recovery happens.[20]

DISASTER PLANNING/ALL-HAZARD PREPAREDNESS

The medical management of patients injured as a result of an intentional or accidental radiation exposure is complex. Preparing a response for unexpected disasters is known as all-hazard preparedness. A hazards vulnerability analysis examines which accidents are possible, which are most likely to occur, and what assets are required for each event. Once these factors are correctly identified then a needs-based assessment can be used to prioritize resources to best cover each of these potential hazards. A well-prepared ICU disaster response plan should address all 4 phases: mitigation, preparedness, response, and recovery. Key to a successful radiation event response is an accurate risk assessment. Specifically, what is the likelihood and expected impact of each event given your location, local, and regional resources. Is there a nuclear power plant in your area, what types of nuclear materials are stored, transported, and used in industry, medicine, and research in your region? Identifying the radiation hazards in your area will allow you to optimize your emergency management plan and use appropriate drill scenarios to best prepare your facility for these types of disasters. Local centers of excellence (eg, bone marrow transplant centers) along with regional and national resources available for assistance should be identified and included in emergency response plans[4,33,34] (see **Box 1**). The National Marrow Donor Program and the American Society for Blood and Marrow Transplantation have established the Radiation Injury Treatment Network, a consortium of transplant centers and other facilities dedicated to providing assistance with the response to disasters involving ionizing radiation.[35] Likewise the European Group for Blood and Marrow Transplantation has established a similar network in Europe.

> **Box 1**
> **A selection of available online resources**
>
> US Radiologic Emergency Response Resources:
>   Armed Forces Radiobiology Research Institute (AFRRI) Bethesda, Md, Medical Radiobiology
>   Advisory Team (MRAT), U.S. Department of Defense. Web site: www.afrri.usuhs.mil.
>   Centers for Disease Control and Prevention (CDC), Atlanta, Ga, Emergency Preparedness and
>   Response. Web site: www.bt.cdc.gov.
>   Radiation Emergency Assistance Center/Training Site (REAC/TS), Oak Ridge, Tenn, U.S.
>   Department of Energy. Web site: www.orise.orau.gov/reacts.
>   Radiation Event Medical Management (REMM), U.S. Department of Health and Human
>   Services. Web site: www.remm.nlm.gov.
>   Radiation Injury Treatment Network. http://www.ritn.net/
>   WHO Radiation Emergency Medical Preparedness and Assistance Network (REMPAN) https://
>   www.who.int/ionizing_radiation/a_e/rempan/en/

SUMMARY

Although unlikely, radiologic and nuclear events should be considered when formulating disaster response plans for the ICU. The medical management of this group of patients is complex and resource intensive. Careful clinical evaluation and an accurate assessment of individual radiation dose is critical in accurate triage, and allows optimization of resources to do most good for most casualties. Knowledge of local centers of excellence and regional and national resources is vital to the successful management of these patients.

ACKNOWLEDGMENTS

The views expressed herein are those of the author(s) and do not necessarily reflect the official policy or position of the Department of the Navy, Department of Defense, or the U.S. Government.

REFERENCES

1. Coeytaux K, Bey E, Christensen D, et al. Reported radiation overexposure accidents worldwide, 1980-2013: a systematic review. Plos One 2015;10(3).
2. Christodouleas J, Forrest R, Ainsley C, et al. Short-term and long-term health risks of nuclear-power-plant accidents. New Engl J Med 2011;364(24):2334–41.
3. Woodruff C, Alt L, Forcino D, et al. Radiological events and their consequences. Fort Detrick (MD): Bordon Institute; 2012.
4. Gale R, Armitage J. Are we prepared for nuclear terrorism? New Engl J Med 2018;378(13):1246–54.
5. Jefferson RD, Goans RE, Blain PG, et al. Diagnosis and treatment of polonium poisoning. Clin Toxicol 2009;47(5):379–92.
6. Madrid J. Radiological considerations in medical operations. Fort Detrick (MD): Bordon Institute; 2012.
7. (REAC/TS) REACTS. The medical aspects of radiation incidents. 4th edition. Oak Ridge (TN): Oak Ridge Institute for Science and Education; 2017. Available at: www.orise.orau.gov/reacts. Accessed February 1,2019.
8. Flynn D, Goans R. Acute radiation syndrome in humans. Fort Detrick (MD): Bordon Institute; 2012.
9. Christensen DM, Iddins CJ, Sugarman SL. Ionizing radiation injuries and illnesses. Emerg Med Clin North America 2014;32(1):245–65.

10. Wolbarst AB, Wiley AL, Nemhauser JB, et al. Medical response to a major radiologic emergency: a primer for medical and public health practitioners. Radiology 2010;254(3):660–77.

11. Yoo J, Jin Y. Establishment of criteria for skin decontamination in a radiation emergency. Health Phys 2018;115(3):369–74.

12. REMM Radiation Emergency Medical Management. US department of health and human services. Available at: www.remm.nlm.gov/. Accessed Feb 1, 2019.

13. REMM. REMM Radiation Emergency Medical Management. US department of health and human services. Available at: www.remm.nlm.gov/. Accessed Feb 1, 2019.

14. (AFRRI) AFRRI. Biodosimetry tools. Available at: https://www.usuhs.edu/afrri/biodosimetrytools. Accessed Feb 1, 2019.

15. Sproull M, Camphausen K. State-of-the-art advances in radiation biodosimetry for mass casualty events involving radiation exposure. Radiat Res 2016;186(5):423–35.

16. Rea M, Gougelet R, Nicolalde R, et al. Proposed triage categories for large-scale radiation incidents using high-accuracy biodosimetry methods. Health Phys 2010;98(2):136–44.

17. Swartz H, Williams B, Nicolalde R, et al. Overview of biodosimetry for management of unplanned exposures to ionizing radiation. Radiat Measurements 2011; 46(9):742–8.

18. Demidenko E, Williams B, Swartz H. Radiation dose prediction using data on time to emesis in the case of nuclear terrorism. Radiat Res 2009;171(3):310–9.

19. Blumenthal DJ, Sugarman SL, Christensen DM, et al. Role of dicentric analysis in an overarching biodosimetry strategy for use following a nuclear detonation in an urban environment. Health Phys 2014;106(4):516–22.

20. Flynn D, Goans R. Triage and treatment of radiation and combined-injury mass casualties. Fort Detrick (MD): Borden Institute, Office of the Surgeon General; 2012.

21. Singh V, Garcia M, Seed T. A review of radiation countermeasures focusing on injury-specific medicinals and regulatory approval status: part II. Countermeasures for limited indications, internalized radionuclides, emesis, late effects, and agents demonstrating efficacy in large animals with or without FDA IND status. Int J Radiat Biol 2017;93(9):870–84.

22. Singh V, Seed T. A review of radiation countermeasures focusing on injury-specific medicinals and regulatory approval status: part I. Radiation subsyndromes, animal models and FDA-approved countermeasures. Int J Radiat Biol 2017;93(9):851–69.

23. Kazzi Z, Buzzell J, Bertelli L, et al. Emergency department management of patients internally contaminated with radioactive material. Emerg Med Clin North America 2015;33(1):179–+.

24. Smith T, Bohlke K, Lyman G, et al. Recommendations for the use of WBC growth factors: American Society of Clinical Oncology Clinical Practice Guideline Update. J Clin Oncol 2015;33(28):3199–212.

25. Dainiak N. Rationale and recommendations for treatment of radiation injury with cytokines. Health Phys 2010;98(6):838–42.

26. Reeves G. Overview of use of G-CSF and GM-CSF in the treatment of acute radiation injury. Health Phys 2014;106(6):699–703.

27. Dainiak N. Medical management of acute radiation syndrome and associated infections in a high-casualty incident. J Radiat Res 2018;59(suppl_2):ii54–64.

28. Freifeld A, Bow E, Sepkowitz K, et al. Clinical practice guideline for the use of antimicrobial agents in neutropenic patients with cancer: 2010 update by the Infectious Diseases Society of America. Clin Infect Dis 2011;52(4):E56–93.
29. Waselenko J, MacVittie T, Blakely W, et al. Medical management of the acute radiation syndrome: recommendations of the Strategic National Stockpile Radiation Working Group. Ann Intern Med 2004;140(12):1037–51.
30. Dainiak N, Gent R, Carr Z, et al. Literature review and global consensus on management of acute radiation syndrome affecting nonhematopoietic organ systems. Disaster Med Public Health Preparedness 2011;5(3):183–201.
31. Dainiak N, Gent R, Carr Z, et al. First global consensus for evidence-based management of the hematopoietic syndrome resulting from exposure to ionizing radiation. Disaster Med Public Health Preparedness 2011;5(3):202–12.
32. Rosas-Palma C, Liland A, Jerstad AN, et al, editors. TMT handbook. Triage, monitoring and treatment of people exposed to ionizing radiation following a malevolent act. Østerås, Norway: Norwegian Radiation Protection Authority; 2009. Available at: https://www.remm.nlm.gov/tmt-handbook-20091.pdf. Accessed February 14, 2019.
33. DiCarlo A, Maher C, Hick J, et al. Radiation injury after a nuclear detonation: medical consequences and the need for scarce resources allocation. Disaster Med Public Health Preparedness 2011;5:S32–44.
34. Dainiak N, Skudlarska B, Albanese J. Local, regional and national responses for medical management of a radiological/nuclear incident. Dose-Response 2013; 11(1):121–9.
35. Case C. Radiation injury treatment network (R): preparedness through a coalition of cancer centers. Health Phys 2016;111(2):145–8.

Chemical Agents in Disaster
Care and Management in the Intensive Care Unit

Rashmi Mishra, MD[a],*, James Geiling, MD, MPH[b,c]

KEYWORDS

- Chemical agents • Chemical attack • Intensive care unit
- Chemical agents of warfare • Chemical weapons of mass destruction • Nerve agents
- Vesicants • Blood agents

KEY POINTS

- Chemical agents of warfare are commonly classified into lung agents, nerve agents, vesicants, and blood agents.
- Key principles of management in the intensive care unit include supportive care and early administration of antidote.
- Aggressive intensive care can lead to significant recovery among patients, even with those with seemingly poor prognosis.
- Hospitals may be overwhelmed in the event of a chemical attack. A plan for emergency response must be established in each hospital to deal with such an emergency.
- Managing critically ill patients exposed to chemical agents requires coordination with other prehospital and emergency department team members in order to ensure the safety of critical care providers.

INTRODUCTION

Chemical agents have been used in warfare for many centuries. Their use during World War 1 and in early 1900s led to the Geneva Convention of 1925. This treaty banned the use of chemical agents of warfare (CAW).[1] However, CAW have still been sporadically used throughout the twentieth century.[2–4] The Chemical Weapons Convention went

Disclosure Statement: The authors do not have a financial relationship with a commercial entity that has an interest in the subject of the article. The opinions and assertions contained herein are those of the authors and do not necessarily reflect the views or position of the Department of Veterans Affairs, the Geisel School of Medicine at Dartmouth, or Penn Highlands Healthcare. No financial support was used for this article.
[a] The Lung Center, Penn Highlands Healthcare, 100 Hospital Avenue, DuBois, PA 15801, USA;
[b] Geisel School of Medicine at Dartmouth, Hanover, NH 03755, USA; [c] Medical Service, VA Medical Center, White River Junction, VT 05009, USA
* Corresponding author.
E-mail address: rashmi_mishra1987@yahoo.com

into effect in 1997, which prohibits the development, production, acquisition, stockpiling, retention, transfer, or use of chemical weapons by signatory states.[5] Despite these measures, CAW have emerged as a growing threat because raw materials for their production is cheap, widely available, and difficult to detect. Critical care providers will play an important part in managing patients in the event of a chemical attack. A significant number of patients may require management in the intensive care unit (ICU) depending on the dose, time, and concentration of exposure to CAW in such an event.[6] Intensivists must familiarize themselves with the clinical effects and management principles of exposure to different chemical agents.

Classification of Chemical Agents

Classification of CAW is based on their mechanisms of action and physiologic effects. The most common classification is as follows:

- Lung agents
- Nerve agents
- Vesicants
- Blood agents[6]

General Principles

The basic principle of ICU management during a chemical attack is providing supportive care and early administration of antidotes. The symptoms and signs after exposure to a CAW can vary depending on the route, dose, duration as well as the concentration of exposure and rapidity of decontamination in the field. Some patients who seem clinically stable initially may decompensate later on, and therefore, need closer monitoring (eg, lung agents). The other end of the spectrum is that even patients with seemingly poor prognosis may recover completely. Importantly, not all patients will have received appropriate and necessary decontamination in the prehospital setting. Patients who arrive without this care may put health care providers in the emergency department and ICU at risk for chemical contamination, causing a hospital to be easily overwhelmed in the event of such an attack.[7] A planned emergency response should be in place in every hospital to deal with chemical attacks.[6]

LUNG AGENTS

Lung or "choking" agents cause acute lung injury after inhalation. Patients exposed to lung agents are very likely to require critical care management. The most common chemicals in this category are phosgene and chlorine.

Gases like ammonia or hydrogen chloride, which are very water soluble, affect the eyes and upper airway mucous membranes. Chlorine, which is a moderately water-soluble gas, affects the upper airway to some extent, but also damages the alveoli. Phosgene, on the other hand, which is very slightly water soluble, primarily affects the alveoli. The gases affecting primarily upper airways are classified as "centrally acting agents." Those that primarily affect the alveoli or lung parenchyma are classified as "peripherally acting agents."[7,8]

Exposure to centrally acting agents may cause severe laryngospasm (and possibly death). Further exposure of the mucous membranes can lead to burning sensation in eyes, conjunctival erythema, rhinorrhea, watering of eyes, hoarseness of voice, sore throat, dysphagia, coughing and wheezing, and tightness in the chest. Long-term airway narrowing may occur depending on the dose and duration of exposure.[8]

Peripherally acting agents can cause symptoms after a latency period of 30 minutes to up to 72 hours depending on the exposure. The patient will develop symptoms of cough, dyspnea, and chest tightness after the latency period. Exposure to these agents may lead to noncardiogenic pulmonary edema, diffuse bronchoalveolar injury, bronchospasm, adult respiratory distress syndrome (ARDS), and life-threatening respiratory failure.[8–10] Close monitoring of patients exposed to peripherally acting agents is necessary for early recognition and treatment of these delayed signs and symptoms. Early discharge without close monitoring may lead to delay in care and poor outcomes.[8]

Chest imaging findings in these patients may appear up to 24 hours after the onset of symptoms. These symptoms include alveolar infiltrates, bilateral consolidation, noncardiogenic pulmonary edema, and parenchymal densities.[11,12] Diagnosis should be based on the history of exposure and the clinical presentation because there are no specific laboratory abnormalities that are diagnostic.

Management

Management of patients exposed to inhaled phosgene and chlorine is essentially supportive. No specific antidotes exist. Aggressive early supportive care is required in these patients.

Decontamination (if not already performed in the field) should be performed by washing the patient with soap and water for 3 to 5 minutes and flushing the eyes with normal saline. Exertion should be minimized during transport and hospitalization because this may exacerbate the toxicity of lung agents.[8]

Early intubation and mechanical ventilation may be required for severe laryngospasm, management of pulmonary edema, and severe bronchospasm. Management of increased secretions with frequent suctioning will also be facilitated by early intubation.[6,13] Orotracheal intubation under direct visualization may be warranted in view of edema and laryngospasm that may be present. Lung protective strategy should be used during management of mechanical ventilation because of the high incidence of acute lung injury and ARDS.[6,14] In animal models, lung protective strategy and positive end expiratory pressure appear beneficial, improving oxygenation and overall mortality.[15,16]

Animal models suggest that early initiation of continuous positive airway pressure after 1 hour of exposure and before development of overt clinical signs may improve survival.[17] However, human data do not exist to support this.

Bronchodilator therapy with nebulized β2 agonist can be used for treatment of bronchospasm. Nebulized ipratropium may be added to the regimen. Systemic corticosteroids may be useful in the treatment of severe bronchospasm based on animal studies; however, there are no strong human data to support this practice.[18,19] Prophylactic antibiotics are not warranted. However, evidence for infection should prompt judicious use of antibiotics. Bacterial superinfection may occur 3 to 5 days after exposure. Fevers, elevated white blood cell count, and thick, purulent sputum should prompt the physician to obtain cultures and initiate empiric antibiotics.[8] The data for use of N-acetylcysteine (NAC) for phosgene-induced lung injury are conflicting.[20,21] Ibuprofen has shown some efficacy in preventing phosgene-induced lung injury in animal models.[22] Both NAC and ibuprofen do not have human data to support their routine clinical use. There are case reports suggesting use of high-volume hemofiltration if conservative measures fail; however, no trials exist to support its use.[23]

Most individuals who survive phosgene or chlorine exposure will recover completely with no long-term effects.[8,24]

NERVE AGENTS

Nerve agents are the most toxic among the CAW. They are clear and colorless in their pure state. When diluted in water, they are mostly tasteless as well. Hence, these are very difficult to detect.

All nerve agents are organophosphorus compounds. They inhibit acetylcholinesterase at cholinergic receptor sites in the central and peripheral nervous systems as well as red blood cells and butyrylcholinesterase in the plasma.[25] Acetylcholine thus accumulates at muscarinic and nicotinic receptors in the central nervous system and neuromuscular junctions of the peripheral nervous system. The clinical manifestations of nerve agents result from the cholinergic overstimulation. Although the symptoms are similar to those produced by organophosphate insecticides, nerve agents can be up to 1000 times more toxic.[26] The term "nerve agents" is given to these compounds because of their significantly higher nicotinic symptoms than insecticides.[27]

The originally developed compounds from Germany are designated as the "G" series of nerve agents. The G series nerve agents include GA (Tabun), GB (Sarin), GD (Soman), and GF (no common name). These are most toxic when inhaled, although they can be absorbed through skin abrasions, the eyes, and the gut, if ingested. The "V" series of agents are better absorbed through the skin than the "G" agents. The V series nerve agents include VE, VG, VM, and VX (most well known).[27]

Inhalation of nerve agent vapors creates symptoms within seconds to minutes after exposure and reaches maximum severity within minutes. Dermal exposure can lead to symptoms within 2 to 30 minutes with severe exposure; however, symptoms may be delayed by up to 18 hours with mild to moderate exposure.[26] The commonly known acronym "SLUDGE": salivation, lacrimation, urination, defecation, gastric distress, and emesis, can be used to remember the muscarinic effects of nerve agents. "DUMBELS": diarrhea, urination, miosis, bradycardia/bronchorrhea/bronchospasm, emesis, lacrimation, salivation/secretion/sweating, is another acronym to remember the symptoms. The "Killer B's": bronchorrhea, bronchoconstriction, bradycardia can be used to remember the symptoms that require immediate intervention.[27,28]

Signs and symptoms of each organ system owing to nerve agent exposure are summarized in **Table 1**.

In the event of a significant high-dose exposure, minor symptoms may not be evident. Patients may present with loss of consciousness, central apnea, and seizures following exposure. The dose range for minor to fatal symptoms is very narrow as well, causing most patients to present with severe symptoms.[25]

The Peradeniya Organophosphorus Poisoning scale (POP scale) was created in Sri Lanka to assess severity of organophosphate poisoning. Although not validated in nerve agent poisonings, it can help with prognostication. The POP scale, outlined in **Table 2**, correlates with death, the need for intubation, and the dosage of atropine required. None of the patients with a score less than 3 died in the study. Of course, clinical assessment by the bedside physician takes precedence over any created scale.[27,32]

Diagnosis of nerve agent poisoning should be based on clinical symptoms. Confirmatory tests consisting of erythrocyte cholinesterase activity is neither widely available nor useful in predicting the severity of symptoms. There may be elevation of creatine kinase and lactic acid. Sarin gas can also cause laboratory abnormalities suggestive of hypoadrenalism.[30]

Supportive Care

Decontamination is a key step in the treatment of any CAW exposure, if not performed in the field. Decontamination after life-saving measures and administration of

Table 1
Effects of exposure to nerve agents

Organ System	Effects of Exposure to Nerve Agents
Pulmonary	Bronchorrhea, bronchoconstriction Cough, dyspnea Wheezing
Cardiac	Bradycardia (cholinergic overstimulation) First-, second-, and third-degree heart blocks Nicotinic receptor–mediated tachycardia Prolongation of QTc interval; Torsades de pointes Elevated blood pressures
Central nervous system (CNS; peripheral and central)	Muscle fasciculations Muscle weakness, muscle paralysis (including the diaphragm) Profuse sweating Seizures, status epilepticus Loss of consciousness Insomnia, irritability, depression, mild confusion, anxiety, memory impairment (mild) Centrally mediated apnea Depression of medullary function (Sarin)
Ocular	Miosis Ocular pain Lacrimation Blurred vision Injected conjunctiva
Gastrointestinal	Nausea, vomiting Abdominal cramping Diarrhea
Ear, nose, throat	Rhinorrhea Salivation

Data from Refs.[1,25,26,29–31]

Table 2
The Peradeniya Organophosphorus Poisoning scale

Pupil size	>2 mm	0
	<2 mm	1
	Pinpoint	2
Respiratory rate	<20/min	0
	>20/min	1
	>20/min with central cyanosis	2
Heart rate	>60/min	0
	41–60/min	1
	<40/min	2
Fasciculation	None	0
	Present, generalized, or continuous	1
	Present, generalized, and continuous	2
Level of consciousness	Conscious and rational	0
	Impaired response to verbal commands	1
	No response to verbal commands	2
Seizures	Absent	0
	Present	1

0 to 3, mild poisoning; 4 to 7, moderate poisoning; 8 to 11, severe poisoning.
From Senanayake N, de Silva HJ, Karalliedde L. A scale to assess severity in organophosphorous intoxication: POP scale. Hum ExpToxicol. 1993;12:297–299; with permission.

antidotes are essential to prevent prolonged exposure to nerve agents. Removal of contaminated clothing, prolonged washing of the patient with soap and water, and rinsing the eyes with water should be sufficient.[7,25] Personal protective equipment as per OSHA guidelines and respective hospital guidelines should be worn by the staff during this step.[33] Decontamination must occur before transfer to the ICU to prevent contamination.

The initial management of all nerve agent exposures consists of the traditional "ABCs" of resuscitation: airway, breathing, and circulation support. Death from exposure to nerve agents is primarily due to respiratory failure.[34] Hence, airway management and ventilatory support are critical steps in the management of these patients. Endotracheal intubation may be required owing to decreased level of consciousness, seizures as well as generalized weakness in addition to respiratory failure, bronchorrhea, and bronchospasm.[6] Nausea and vomiting may further complicate the intubation process. An anticipated difficult airway and high risk for aspiration owing to a full stomach are recommended.[26]

Mechanical ventilation in these patients can be difficult because of significant bronchospasm and copious secretions leading to high airway pressures.[26] Endotracheal intubation is preferred over a laryngeal mask airway if bronchospasm and copious secretions are present.[35] Nebulized ipratropium can be used for the treatment of bronchospasm.[25] Neuromuscular blocking agents should be avoided to prevent compounding the effects of nerve agents.[36] Mechanical ventilation support is normally much shorter in nerve agent poisonings than for organophosphate poisonings. Organophosphates in the form of pesticides can get sequestered in the body owing to higher fat solubility and lower rate of metabolism. Most patients with nerve gas poisonings will require ventilator support for less than 24 hours as opposed to those with pesticide poisoning, who may require mechanical ventilation for longer periods.[26]

Antidote

Atropine is the principal antidote for nerve agents. It works through competitive antagonism against the nerve agent.[27] It blocks acetylcholine receptor sites, most effectively at muscarinic sites. Thus, atropine prevents the anticholinergic effects of the nerve agents, which lead to decreased bronchoconstriction, bronchorrhea, salivation, and abdominal smooth muscle cramps. Primarily used to decrease airway secretions, atropine is administered at a standard dosing of 2 mg, intramuscularly or intravenously, every 5 to 10 minutes titrated to secretions in the endotracheal tube.[26,34] Adults can require 10 to 20 mg of atropine in the first hour to control secretions. In cases of severe poisoning, an initial dose of 6 mg may be used.[26] Oxygen should be administered to correct hypoxemia before atropine administration to prevent precipitation of ventricular fibrillation.[37,38] Miosis and ocular pain may be treated with topical tropicamide.[27,34]

"Oximes" are another major antidote for nerve agents. They work by removing the phosphyl moiety of the phosphorylated enzyme (organophosphate-inhibited cholinesterase), thus reactivating the enzyme. Oximes must be administered early before the bond between the agent and enzyme "ages," making the bond irreversible and renders them ineffective. The "aging" process may take as little as 2 minutes with soman and up to 3 to 4 hours for sarin.[26] 2-PAM (pralidoxime chloride), dosed at 15 to 25 mg per kilogram or 1 to 2 g if given intravenously over 20 to 30 minutes, works on the nicotinic sites and helps improve muscle strength. The initial dose may be followed by an infusion of 200 to 500 mg per hour, if necessary.[27] An initial 2-g load followed by 1 g per hour for 48 hours was shown to decrease atropine requirements and duration of mechanical ventilation in patients poisoned by organophosphate pesticides in 1 study.[39] Severe hypertension after administration of pralidoxime chloride may occur and can be reversed by a 5-mg intravenous infusion of phentolamine.[34,40]

The military uses diazepam for the management of seizures.[34] In the hospital setting, intensivists may use any benzodiazepine for the treatment of seizures.[27,41] Providers must carefully monitor patients for signs of ventilatory failure following the administration of benzodiazepines. Dexmedetomidine was recently studied in the treatment of benzodiazepine refractory nerve agent–induced status epilepticus and found to be effective.[42]

VESICANTS

This class of CAW, also known as "blister agents," is principally divided into 3 categories: mustards, arsenicals, and urticants. Urticants (characterized by phosgene oxime) are not a real vesicant and causes hives/urticaria rather than blisters.[43] This section will not address urticants.

Vesicants most commonly refer to sulfur mustard (bis-[2-chloroethyl] sulfide), which is commonly referred to as "mustard" because it classically smells like onion, garlic, or mustard.[43] Sulfur mustard is a dense, yellow-to-brown, oily liquid with low volatility and a freezing point of 14.4 C. Lewisite (an organoarsenic vesicant) is also an oily liquid, although more volatile than sulfur mustard with a freezing point of 0.48 F. Exposures to vesicants can occur via skin contact, inhalation of vapors, or ingestion of the agent.[44,45]

The mechanism of action of mustard is proposed to be through alkylation of DNA leading to breaking of strands. Another hypothesis is its reaction with glutathione, a free oxygen radical scavenger, leading to its depletion. These both can lead to cell death. Arsenics like lewisite, on the other hand, inhibit enzymes with sulfhydryl group, leading to NADPH and glutathione depletion, leading to cell death or necrosis.[43,45]

Vesicants can damage the skin they contact. Nitrogen will produce erythema within 4 to 8 hours of exposure, progressing to vesicles 2 to 18 hours later. Lesions are thin-walled, initially translucent, and vary in size from 5 mm to 5 cm. Later in the course, the lesions become yellow and can coagulate. The fluid in the bulla does not contain vesicant, and hence, is not harmful to health care providers. Mustard-induced bullae may take weeks to months to heal. Lewisite causes pain and blister formation within minutes of exposure but tends to heal faster than mustard-induced bullae.[43,45]

Mustard coming in contact with eyes can produce conjunctivitis, blepharospasm, corneal vesicles and sloughing, corneal pannus formation, corneal ulcerations, keratitis, and possibly blindness if the pannus covers the visual axis. Lewisite exposure causes intense irritation and pain with blepharospasm, and hence, further severe injury from it is less common.[43,46]

Mustard vapor inhalation leads to damage of the respiratory tract, starting with upper airways at lower dosages to lower airways with higher dosage. Exposure to high dosages can lead to severe inflammation, necrosis, and sloughing of mucous membranes, leading to pseudomembrane formation, which may obstruct the lower airways. Asthma, laryngospasm, acute and chronic bronchitis, tracheobronchial stenosis, pulmonary fibrosis, and bronchiolitis obliterans are other reported pulmonary complications.[47,48] Hemorrhagic bronchitis can be seen with exposure to high concentrations. Lewisite causes similar injury patterns and can lead to pulmonary edema with exposure to large concentrations.[43,45]

Nausea, vomiting, pancytopenia, and sepsis owing to leukopenia and breakdown of skin and mucosae have been reported with higher doses of mustard exposure.[49]

Lewisite does not have these gastrointestinal and hematologic effects, but can cause capillary leak, hemoconcentration, and hypotension in high-dose exposures.[45]

Supportive Care

Decontamination prevents further injuries to the patients. Again, it should ideally be performed before hospital admission to prevent exposure of health care workers to these vesicants.

Topical silver sulfadiazine and topical antibiotics are recommended for topical applications on denuded skin. Similar to burn patients, pain control, fluid replacement, and prevention of infections are important among these patients. Application of deferoxamine or zinc oxide may also be beneficial.[50] Skin grafts and reconstructive surgeries may be required in some patients because of the longer healing times of these wounds. Patients who have ocular exposure should initially undergo irrigation; then further treatment with mydriasis, topical antibiotics, daily irrigation to remove inflammatory debris, and consultation with an ophthalmologist. Topical steroids may be helpful.[43,46]

Respiratory care is mostly supportive. Bronchodilators for asthmalike symptoms, and corticosteroids in bronchodilator-nonresponsive patients may be used. Early intubation and ventilator support should be considered before development of severe laryngospasm. Endotracheal intubation also allows for frequent suctioning of inflammatory debris. Bronchoscopy may be necessary to remove pseudomembrane fragments from the airway. Chronic, progressive tracheobronchial stenosis was reported in 10% of Iranian casualties. Patients with tracheobronchial stenosis will require frequent bronchoscopies and dilation.[43,51]

For systemic toxicity, nonsteroidal anti-inflammatory drugs and granulocyte colony-stimulating factors may be considered in addition to conservative measures.[52]

Antidote

Dimercaprol or British anti-lewisite (BAL) is an antidote for lewisite exposure. BAL binds to the arsenic of lewisite more strongly than do tissue enzymes, thereby displacing lewisite from the cellular receptor sites reducing the systemic effects of the lewisite exposure. It can be given intramuscularly. Topical formulations for cutaneous and ocular exposure are not available in the United States.[43] No antidote for mustard exists.

Although the acute mortality from these agents is low, recovery times are prolonged and associated with high morbidity. Significant health care resources are expended in the management of the sequelae of exposure among these patients.

BLOOD AGENTS

"Blood agents" and cyanide are agents that work by causing "histotoxic anoxia."[53] Cyanide binds to the active site of cytochrome c oxidase, which leads to the inability of cells to use oxygen to produce adenosine triphosphate (ATP). Hence, the cells are forced to convert to anaerobic metabolism. Cyanide can be used as an agent of mass destruction in 2 chemical forms: hydrogen cyanide and cyanogen chloride. The volatility of cyanide makes it difficult to weaponize. Cyanide may exist in gaseous form or as a colorless liquid. Classically, it has the smell of "bitter almonds," although about half the population cannot identify this odor.[53,54]

The clinical manifestations of cyanide poisoning are due to the tissue hypoxia it causes. Following inhalation, the effects of cyanide can be rapid, within 15 seconds, but may take up to 30 minutes following ingestion. The clinical effects of cyanide poisoning are summarized in **Table 3**.

Table 3 Clinical effects of cyanide	
Organ	**Effect**
CNS	Loss of consciousness Convulsions Decreased awareness
Metabolic	Lactic acidosis, anion gap metabolic acidosis Decreased ATP

Pulmonary	Initial:
	  Tachypnea, increased minute ventilation
	Late:
	  Apnea

Cardiac	Initial:
	  Hypertension
	  Arrhythmias
	Late:
	  Hypotension
	  Decreased cardiac output
	  Shock

Ophthalmology	Late: Dilated pupils with variable reactivity
Gastrointestinal	Nausea Vomiting

Data from Baskin SI, Brewer TG. Cyanide poisoning, in Sidell FR, Takafuji ET, Franz DR (eds): Medical Aspects of Chemical and Biological Warfare, in Zajtchuk R, Bellamy RF (eds): Textbook of Military Medicine, Part I: Warfare, Weaponry and the Casualty. Washington, DC, United States Department of the Army, Office of the Surgeon General and Borden Institute, 1997: 271-286 and Toxicological profile for cyanide. U.S. Department of Health and Human Services. Public Health Service. Agency For Toxic Substances And Disease Registry. July 2006. Available at: https://permanent.access.gpo.gov/gpo29203/tp8-c1-b.pdf. Accessed Feb 24, 2019

Late signs of cyanide poisoning include dilated unresponsive pupils, which portend a poor prognosis. Eventually, the patients develop apnea and cardiac dysrhythmias followed by death from cardiac arrest.[53] The survival rate after onset of arrhythmias is very low at about 3%.[55]

Intensivists will likely treat patients with mild to moderate poisoning who survive till they reach an ICU or severe poisoning cases whereby the antidote was given early in the field. The classic signs pointing to cyanide poisoning in the ICU (apart from history) are bright red venous blood, unexplained significant lactic acidosis, and significant dyspnea in the absence of cyanosis. Treatment of cyanide poisoning should include early supportive care and administration of antidote simultaneously.

Supportive Care

Supportive measures include establishment of airway for altered level of consciousness, seizures, hypoxemia, hypercapnia, or significant metabolic acidosis. Administration of 100% oxygen is helpful by decreasing CO_2 levels. Vasopressor support may be required if hemodynamics are compromised.[6] Seizures should be managed with benzodiazepines. Standard antiarrhythmic medications should be used for the treatment of arrhythmias, although arrhythmias portend a poor prognosis.[53] Hyperbaric oxygen may be helpful in severe poisoning cases poisoning.[56] Sodium bicarbonate can be considered for treatment of severe acidosis with monitoring of arterial blood gases.[53,57]

Antidote

Sodium nitrite and sodium thiosulfate

This combination detoxifies and excretes the cyanide. Initial sodium nitrite administration (300 mg in 10-mL diluents given over 2–4 minutes) leads to formation of methemoglobin. Cyanide binds preferentially to the ferric ion site of methemoglobin, thereby removing cyanide from the cytochrome c. Because sodium nitrite produces methemoglobin and can cause hypotension, methemoglobin levels and blood pressure should be monitored during the therapy and nitrite held if deemed necessary until hypotension resolves or elevated methemoglobin levels decrease to therapeutic levels (<10%). Following this, administration of sodium thiosulfate (12.5 g of sodium thiosulfate in 50 mL of diluent administered at 3–5 mL per minute intravenously) acts as a substrate for rhodanese, thereby converting cyanide to thiocyanide, which is then excreted in the urine. The combination is an effective antidote, if given before onset of cardiac arrest.[56] Animal models suggest intramuscular injections of sodium nitrite and sodium thiosulfate may also be sufficient.[58]

Hydroxocobalamin

An alternative treatment option for cyanide poisoning is the more expensive hydroxocobalamin (5 g infused over 15 minutes). Hydroxocobalamin, a precursor of vitamin B12, binds with cyanide to form cyanocobalamin, which is then excreted in the urine.[59] It has been associated with oxalate nephropathy and acute kidney injury, although there does not appear to be sufficient evidence to discourage its use.[60,61]

SUMMARY

Intensivists are very likely to be involved in the care of patients exposed to CAW. Aggressive supportive care is warranted in most cases. Understanding clinical features, basic management principles, and prognostic markers is important. Many severely ill patients may make full recovery. The other end of the spectrum is the significant number of "worried well" who do not require any significant treatments. Hence, judicious use of available resources for the patients requiring intensive care to recover is essential. Intensivists must be prepared to deal with the recognition, medical management, and psychological trauma of casualties resulting from CAW.

REFERENCES

1. 1925 Geneva Protocol. Available at: https://www.un.org/disarmament/wmd/bio/1925-geneva-protocol/. Accessed March 2, 2019.
2. Smart JK. History of chemical and biological warfare: an American perspective. In: Sidell FR, Takafuji ET, Franz DR, editors. Medical aspects of chemical and biological warfare, in Zajtchuk R, Bellamy RF (editors): Textbook of military medicine, Part I: warfare, Weaponry and the casualty. Washington, DC: United States Department of the Army, Office of the Surgeon General and Borden Institute; 1997. p. 9–86.
3. Okudera H, Morita H, Iwashita T, et al. Unexpected nerve gas exposure in the city of Matsumoto: report of rescue activity in the first sarin gas terrorism. Am J Emerg Med 1997;15(5):527–8.
4. Okumura T, Takasu N, Ishimatsu S, et al. Report on 640 victims of the Tokyo subway sarin attack. Ann Emerg Med 1996;28(2):129–35.
5. Convention on the prohibition of the development, production, stockpiling and use of chemical weapons and on their destruction (chemical weapons convention). Available at: https://www.opcw.org/chemical-weapons-convention. Accessed March 1, 2019.

6. Chalela JA, Burnett T. Chemical terrorism for the intensivist. Mil Med 2012;177(5): 495–500.
7. Okumura T, Suzuki K, Fukuda A, et al. The Tokyo subway sarin attack: disaster management, Part 2: hospital response. Acad Emerg Med 1998;5(6):618–24.
8. Urbanetti JS. Toxic inhalational injury in Sidell FR. In: Takafuji ET, Franz DR, editors. Medical aspects of chemical and biological Warfare,in Zajtchuk R, Bellamy RF (editors): Textbook of military medicine, Part I: warfare, Weaponry and the casualty. Washington, DC: United States Department of the Army, Office of the Surgeon General and Borden Institute; 1997. p. 247–70.
9. Das R, Blanc PD. Chlorine gas exposure and the lung. Toxicol Ind Health 1993; 9:439.
10. Bunting H. The pathology of chlorine gas poisoning. In: Fasciculus on chemical warfare medicine, vol. 2. Washington, DC: Committee on Treatment of Gas Casualties, National Research Council; 1945. p. 24.
11. Prevention and treatment of injury from chemical warfare agents. Med Lett Drugs Ther 2002;44(1121):1–4.
12. Van Sickle D, Wenck MA, Belfiower A, et al. Acute health care effects after exposure to chlorine gas released after a train derailment. Am J Emerg Med 2009; 27:1–7.
13. Baker DJ. Management of respiratory failure in toxic disasters. Resuscitation 1999;42:125–31.
14. The Acute Respiratory Distress Syndrome Network. Ventilation with lower tidal volumes as compared with traditional tidal volumes for acute lung injury and the acute respiratory distress syndrome. N Engl J Med 2000;342:1301–8.
15. Parkhouse DA, Brown RF, Jugg BJ, et al. Protective ventilation strategies in the management of phosgene-induced acute lung injury. Mil Med 2007;172(3): 295–300.
16. Li W, Rosenbruch M, Pauluhn J. Effect of PEEP on phosgene-induced lung edema: pilot study on dogs using protective ventilation strategies. Exp Toxicol Pathol 2015;67(2):109–16.
17. Graham S, Fairhall S, Rutter S, et al. Continuous positive airway pressure: an early intervention to prevent phosgene-induced acute lung injury. Toxicol Lett 2018; 293:120–6.
18. Wang J, Winskog C, Edston E, et al. Inhaled and intravenous corticosteroids both attenuate chlorine gas-induced lung injury in pigs. Acta Anaesthesiol Scand 2005;49(2):183–90.
19. Grainge C, Rice P. Management of phosgene-induced acute lung injury. Clin Toxicol 2010;48:497–508.
20. Sciuto AM, Strickland PT, Kennedy TP, et al. Protective effects of N-acetylcysteine treatment after phosgene exposure in rabbits. Am J Respir Crit Care Med 1995; 151:768.
21. Rendell R, Fairhall R, Graham S, et al. Assessment of N-acetylcysteine as a therapy for phosgene-induced acute lung injury. Toxicol Lett 2018;290:145–52.
22. Sciuto AM, Hurt HH. Therapeutic treatments of phosgene-induced lung injury. Inhal Toxicol 2004;16(8):565–80.
23. Wang L, Wu D, Wang J. Chlorine gas inhalation manifesting with severe acute respiratory distress syndrome successfully treated by high-volume hemofiltration: a case report. Medicine (Baltimore) 2018;97(30):e11708.
24. Russell D, Blaine PG, Rice P. Clinical management of casualties exposed to lung damaging agents: a critical review. Emerg Med J 2006;23(6):421–4.

25. Leikin JB, Thomas RG, Walter FG, et al. A review of nerve agent exposure for the critical care physician. Crit Care Med 2002;30(10):2346–54.
26. Sidell FR. Nerve agents. In: Sidell FR, Takafuji ET, Franz DR, editors. Medical aspects of chemicaland biological warfare, in Zajtchuk R, Bellamy RF (editors): Textbook of military medicine, Part I: warfare, Weaponry and the casualty. Washington, DC: United States Department of the Army,Office of the Surgeon General and Borden Institute; 1997. p. 129–80.
27. Wiener SW, Hoffman RS. Nerve agents: a comprehensive review. J Intensive Care Med 2004;19:22–37.
28. Thomas RG. Chemoterrorism, in nerve agents. In: Walter FB, Klein R, Thomas RG, editors. Advanced Hazmat life support provider manual. 3rd edition. Tucson (AZ): University of Arizona Board of Regents; 2003. p. 302.
29. Chuang FR, Jang SW, Lin JL, et al. QTc prolongation indicates a poor prognosis in patients with organophosphate poisoning. Am J Emerg Med 1996;14(5):451–3.
30. Yanagisawa N, Morita H, Nakajima T. Sarin experiences in Japan; acute toxicity and long-term effects. J Neurol Sci 2006;249:76–85.
31. Liu J, Uchea C, Wright L, et al. Chapter 34 – Chemical warfare agents and the nervous system. In: Gupta RC, editor. Handbook of toxicology of chemical warfare agents. 2nd edition. London: Academic Press; 2015. p. 463–75.
32. Senanayake N, de Silva HJ, Karalliedde L. A scale to assess severity in organophosphorous intoxication: POP scale. Hum Exp Toxicol 1993;12:297–9.
33. Horton DK, Berkowitz Z, Kaye WE. Secondary contamination of ED personnel from hazardous materials events, 1995-2001. Am J Emerg Med 2003;21(3):199–204.
34. Lee EC. Clinical manifestations of sarin nerve gas exposure. JAMA 2003;290(5):659–62.
35. de Jong RH. Nerve gas terrorism: a grim challenge to anesthesiologists. Anesth Analg 2003;96(3):819–25.
36. Cosar A, Kenar L. An anesthesiological approach to nerve agent victims. Mil Med 2006;171(1):7–11.
37. Berkenstadt H, Marganitt B, Atsmon J. Combined chemical and conventional injuries—pathophysiological, diagnostic and therapeutic aspects. Isr J Med Sci 1991;27(11–12):623–6.
38. Marik P, Bowles S. Management of patients exposed to biological and chemical warfare agents. J Int Care Med 2002;17(4):147–61.
39. Pawar KS, Bhoite RR, Pillay CP, et al. Continuous pralidoxime infusion versus repeated bolus injection to treat organophosphorus pesticide poisoning: a randomised controlled trial. Lancet 2006;368(9553):2136–41.
40. Watson A, Opresko D, Young RA, et al. Chapter 9 – Organophosphate nerve agents. In: Gupta RC, editor. Handbook of toxicology of chemical warfare agents. 2nd edition. London: Academic Press; 2015. p. 87–109.
41. McDonough JH Jr, McMonagle J, Copeland T, et al. Comparative evaluation of benzodiazepines for control of soman-induced seizures. Arch Toxicol 1999;73(8–9):473–8.
42. McCarren HS, Arbutus JA, Cherish A, et al. Dexmedetomidine stops benzodiazepine-refractory nerve agent-induced status epilepticus. Epilepsy Res 2018;141:1–12.
43. Sidell FR, Urbanetti JS, Smith WJ, et al. Vesicants. In: Sidell FR, Takafuji ET, Franz DR, editors. Medical aspects of chemical and biological warfare, in Zajtchuk R, Bellamy RF (editors): Textbook of military medicine, Part I: warfare,

Weaponry and the casualty. Washington, DC: United States Department of the Army, Office of the Surgeon General and Borden Institute; 1997. p. 197–228.

44. Medical management guidelines for blister agents: sulfur mustard agent H or HD & sulfur mustard agent HT. Available at: http://www.atsdr.cdc.gov/MHMI/mmg165.pdf. Accessed March 1, 2019.

45. McManus J, Huebner K. Vesicants. Crit Care Clin 2005;21(4):707–18.

46. Safarinejad MR, Moosavi SA, Montazeri B. Ocular injuries caused by mustard gas: diagnosis, treatment, and medical defense. Mil Med 2001;166(1):67–70.

47. Emad A, Rezaian GR. The diversity of the effects of sulfur mustard gas inhalation on respiratory system 10 years after a single, heavy exposure: analysis of 197 cases. Chest 1997;112(3):734–8.

48. Thomason JW, Rice TW, Milstone AP. Bronchiolitis obliterans in a survivor of a chemical weapons attack. JAMA 2003;290(5):598–9.

49. Wattana M, Bey T. Mustard gas or sulfur mustard: an old chemical agent as a new terrorist threat. Prehosp Disaster Med 2009;24(1):19–29.

50. Karayilanoğlu T, Gunhan O, Kenar L, et al. The protective and therapeutic effects of zinc chloride and desferrioxamine on skin exposed to nitrogen mustard. Mil Med 2003;168(8):614–7.

51. Freitag L, Firusian N, Stamatis G, et al. The role of bronchoscopy in pulmonary complications due to mustard gas inhalation. Chest 1991;100(5):1436–41.

52. Anderson DR, Holmes WW, Lee RB, et al. Sulfur mustard-induced neutropenia: treatment with granulocyte colony-stimulating factor. Mil Med 2006;171(5): 448–53.

53. Baskin SI, Brewer TG. Cyanide poisoning. In: Sidell FR, Takafuji ET, Franz DR, editors. Medical aspects of chemical and biological warfare, in Zajtchuk R, Bellamy RF (editors): Textbook of military medicine, Part I: warfare, Weaponry and the casualty. Washington, DC: United States Department of the Army, Office of the Surgeon General and Borden Institute; 1997. p. 271–86.

54. Toxicological profile for cyanide. U.S. Department of health and human Services.-Public health Service.Agency for toxic Substances and Disease Registry. Available at: https://permanent.access.gpo.gov/gpo29203/tp8-c1-b.pdf. Accessed February 24, 2019.

55. Fortin JL, Desmettre T, Manzon C, et al. Cyanide poisoning and cardiac disorders; 161 cases. J Emerg Med 2010;38:467–76.

56. Kales SN, Christiani DC. Acute chemical emergencies. N Engl J Med 2004; 350(8):800–8.

57. Brivet F, Delfraissy JF, Duche M, et al. Acute cyanide poisoning: recovery with non-specific supportive therapy. Intensive Care Med 1983;9(1):33–5.

58. Bebarta VS, Brittain M, Matthew C, et al. Sodium nitrite and sodium thiosulfate are effective against acute cyanide poisoning when administered by intramuscular injection. Ann Emerg Med 2017;69(6):718–25.e4.

59. Thompson JP, Marrs TC. Hydroxocobalamin in cyanide poisoning. Clin Toxicol (Phila) 2012;50:875–85.

60. Legrand M, Michel T, Daudon M, et al. Risk of oxalate nephropathy with the use of cyanide antidote hydroxocobalamin in critically ill burn patients. Intensive Care Med 2016;42(6):1080–1.

61. Mégarbane B. Hydroxocobalamin-attributed risk of oxalate nephropathy: evidence is not sufficient to change the recommended management of cyanide toxicity by fire smoke inhalation. Intensive Care Med 2016;42(7):1197–8.

Anthropogenic Disasters

Michael Powers, MD, LCDR, MC, USN[a],
Michael James Ellett Monson, LCDR[a], Frederic S. Zimmerman, MD[b],
Sharon Einav, MSc, MD[c], David J. Dries, MSE, MD[d],*

KEYWORDS

- Terrorism • Blast injury • Blunt trauma • Penetrating trauma • Stab wounds

KEY POINTS

- Terrorist and criminal activity creating mass-casualty situations typically involves firearms and explosives.
- Resource consumption for acute medical care and rehabilitation is far greater in patients injured by terrorism or other mass-casualty situations.
- Public health interventions advocated for mass-casualty situations based on military experience may not apply uniformly to civilian terrorism because of a differing pattern of injury.

INTRODUCTION

Anthropogenic disasters can broadly be defined as any disaster that is caused by human action or inaction. This is in contrast with natural disasters, which occur without human interference. Anthropogenic disasters range in scope from person-to-person violence to riots, large-scale terrorism, industrial accidents, and full-scale war. Because an all-encompassing review describing all injuries and medical considerations of these events would be too extensive for this publication, this article focuses on the epidemiology and management of the most common types of trauma caused by large-scale terrorist and criminal activity and the initial therapies expected of intensivists. This information is particularly relevant given the number of mass shootings (Orlando, 2016; Las Vegas, 2017; Parkland, 2018), terrorist bombings (Boston, 2013; Paris, 2015; Sri Lanka, 2019), and vehicle-ramming attacks (Nice, 2016) seen in the past few years.

Disclosures: None.
[a] Department of Pulmonary and Critical Care Medicine, Naval Medical Center San Diego, 34800 Bob Wilson Drive, San Diego, CA 92134, USA; [b] Department of Intensive Care, Shaare Zedek Medical Center, 12 Shmuel Bait Street, P.O. Box 3235, Jerusalem 9103102, Israel; [c] Shaare Zedek Medical Center, 12 Shmuel Bait Street, P.O. Box 3235, Jerusalem 9103102, Israel; [d] University of Minnesota, Minneapolis, MN, USA
* Corresponding author. Regions Hospital, Department of Surgery, 640 Jackson Street, #11503C, St Paul, MN 55101.
E-mail address: david.j.dries@healthpartners.com

Crit Care Clin 35 (2019) 647–658
https://doi.org/10.1016/j.ccc.2019.06.002
0749-0704/19/© 2019 Elsevier Inc. All rights reserved.
criticalcare.theclinics.com

Injuries caused by terrorist and criminal activities can largely be grouped into 3 large categories, blast, blunt, and penetrating trauma. Even stab wounds present differently in the setting of terrorism. Although biological, chemical, and radiologic attacks are possible and have been performed (the anthrax letters in the United States in 2001; the release of the nerve agent sarin gas in the Tokyo subway by the Aum Shinrikyu cult in 1995; and the assassination of Alexander Litvinenko by polonium in 2006), these are the exception rather than the rule. Most terrorist and criminal activities that create mass-casualty situations are performed using weapons more readily available, such as firearms and explosives.[1]

Although not considered a terrorist activity, wildfires are often caused by human action. The incidence of wildfires has increased over the past several years and wildfires can have a unique and dramatic impact on public health and property. This natural calamity is briefly discussed in this article.

BLAST TRAUMA

Blast injuries in the United States are not rare. A 20-year retrospective review by Kapur and colleagues[2] identified more than 36,000 explosion incidents, 5931 bomb-related injuries, and 699 bomb-related deaths in the United States between 1983 and 2002. This figure does not include more recent terrorist attacks over the past 17 years, and does not account for military-related injuries. Primary blast injuries to civilians are also expected to harm persons with more medical comorbidities, and the lack of body armor results in significantly more penetrating trauma.[3]

Explosive attacks have repeatedly been shown to be among the most devastating modalities in criminal and terrorist activities. Primary blast injuries result from rapid changes in atmospheric pressure. The high-pressure gases rapidly expand and compress the surrounding medium, usually air, creating a characteristic acceleration-deceleration mechanism that generates the so-called blast wave. Gas-containing organs, especially lungs, are particularly susceptible to injury. Retrospective studies have shown that the victims of terrorist attacks present for medical care with very different wound patterns compared with non–terror-related trauma. When evaluating adults with injuries from terror-related activities, studies have shown that these patients present with injury patterns that are more severe and more widespread compared with trauma outside of terrorism.

An example of how these injuries differ from other forms of trauma was published by Aharonson-Daniel and colleagues.[4] The records of Israeli children injured from terrorist activities over a 2 year period were reviewed and showed a higher incidence of penetrating trauma (54% vs 9%), internal injury to the torso (11% vs 4%), and severe trauma, defined as an increased Injury Severity Score (ISS) greater than 25 (25% vs 3%), but, interestingly, a lower instance of traumatic brain injury compared with non–terror-related injuries (22% vs 44%).[4] Weil and colleagues[5] noted similar findings when comparing terror-related musculoskeletal injuries with motor vehicle accidents in adults. They found a higher ISS and higher rates of polytrauma, amputations, open fractures, and abdominal injuries.

Specific organ systems are injured differently by explosive injury than by other forms of trauma. Bala and colleagues[6] showed a significant difference in the pattern of both abdominal and thoracic injuries of terrorist-related explosions compared with gunshot wounds (GSWs) and blunt force trauma. ISS scores were higher in patients with blast injuries compared with GSW and blunt trauma (34, 18, and 29 respectively). Injury to 3 or more body regions was found in 85.7% of patients with blast injury, compared with 28% of the GSW group and 25.3% of the blunt trauma group. Bowel injury was found in 71.4% of patients with blast injuries, and in those patients 94.4% of those injuries (all but 1 patient) were caused by penetrating shrapnel.[6] More than half (52.7%) of all patients who experienced explosive insults had lung contusions and almost half (45.5%) required chest tube intervention for pneumothorax treatment.[7] Multiple studies have found that patients who incur blast injuries have a significantly higher mortality compared with non–terror-related trauma.[3–6,8]

PENETRATING TRAUMA

The use of firearms, in attacks against both military personnel and civilians, continues to be the primary means of violence used by both criminals and terrorists worldwide, particularly with the invention of the machine gun.[9] The penetrating trauma caused by gun violence continues to be a common part of practice for intensivists.

Recently, several large public initiatives have placed much of the effort to address the loss of life through strong, unidirectional messaging on external hemorrhage control, with a special emphasis on the use of extremity tourniquets. For example, the Hartford Consensus Joint Committee to Create a National Policy to Enhance Survival in Mass Casualty Shooting Events views hemorrhage control as "second only to engaging and defeating the shooter as key to improving the survival of victims of active shooter incidents," describing external hemorrhage control as "the critical step" in eliminating preventable prehospital death.[10,11]

An epidemiologic analysis of large-scale shootings in the United States over the past 10 years has revealed that the injury patterns of these patients is dramatically different from those of patients with blast injury. In addition, new data about penetrating injury secondary to criminal activity question the effectiveness of tourniquets. Smith and colleagues[12] in 2016 performed a review of 12 mass shootings totaling 139 fatalities. They found that 58% of the victims were shot in the head or chest, and only 20% to the extremities. Only 7% of victims had potentially survivable wounds who did not survive, and, of those, 89% of these wounds were to the chest. There were no reported instances of potential survivors exsanguinating from extremity wounds.[12] This finding is in direct contrast with multiple studies of military personnel injured in the current wars in Iraq and Afghanistan that have reported the primary cause of fatalities to be secondary to blast injuries, ranging from 62% to 74%, with only 22% to 23% of injuries secondary to gunshots.[13,14] Based on these demographics, the current campaign favoring the use of tourniquets and hemorrhage control in the civilian setting for prehospital care of mass shootings, which has been advocated by multiple public organizations, including the Hartford Consensus Committee, may not bring about significant improvement in survival for shooting victims.[1,15] Emphasis is still required on rapid control of the airway and appropriate treatment of penetrating trauma to the thorax and abdomen, which cause significantly higher mortality than injuries to the extremities from penetrating trauma.

BLUNT TRAUMA

Blunt trauma that occurs during terrorist and criminal attacks typically occurs secondary to either the collapse of buildings or from automobile ramming. Given the wide availability of automobiles and that using an automobile as a weapon requires a low technical ability, there has been an increase recently of high-profile automobile-related mass casualties in France, Spain, Germany, Sweden, the United Kingdom, Canada, and the United States, prompting concern that this is becoming a preferred method of attack by so-called lone-wolf attackers and minor terrorist cells.[16,17] According to a US Government report, between 2014 and 2017, terrorists performed 18 vehicle-ramming attacks worldwide, resulting in 181 fatalities and 679 injuries.[18]

The injuries sustained from an automobile-versus-pedestrian collision are of a different pattern and far more severe than an automobile-versus-automobile collision because the pedestrian is unprotected. The casualties of intentional automobile attacks seem to have different injury patterns than pedestrians who are accidentally hit by vehicles. One such example of this was shown by Almogy and colleagues,[19] who reviewed the injuries sustained by both groups of victims. The Abbreviated Injury Score is often higher in intentionally injured patients; these patients are more likely to require intubation by emergency medical services; on average they need to undergo more surgical procedures; and they sustain both a higher number and more severe injuries to the head, face, and spine. Overall, patients with intentional vehicle ramming injuries have a higher mortality and are most likely to die from severe head trauma.

Blunt cerebrovascular injury (BCVI) is an evolving topic in the trauma literature. These injuries primarily include injuries to the carotid and vertebral arteries. Although BCVIs occur in 1% to 2% of patients with blunt injury,[20,21] untreated carotid artery injuries are associated with mortalities as high as 28%, with 48% to 58% having permanent severe neurologic deficits.[22,23] The screening modality of choice for this injury is a computed tomographic angiogram (CTA), with a digital subtraction angiogram (DSA) as the confirmatory imaging study.[24] Ruling out false-positives is extremely important because the treatment of choice for surgically inaccessible injuries is full anticoagulation with either heparin or antiplatelet therapy,[25] which should never be performed indiscriminately in patients with trauma. Shahan and colleagues[24] found in a retrospective trial that, by conducting the imaging studies in this order, a definitive diagnosis by DSA led to avoidance of potentially harmful anticoagulation in 45% of patients false-positive on CTA.

One proven method for screening the victims of blunt trauma has been the use of point-of-care ultrasonography (POCUS). The focused assessment with sonography in trauma (FAST) examination has become a standard in the assessment of patients with trauma. This tool has been shown to have utility in detecting life-threatening injuries in patients with blunt trauma.[26] The FAST examination is one of the rapid methods of diagnosing posttraumatic pericardial tamponade and hemoperitoneum.[27,28] In a recent Cochrane Review, the use of POCUS in thoracic and abdominal trauma was examined. Reviewers found a very high sensitivity and specificity with thoracic trauma, but this decreased as abdominal injuries were examined, and the sensitivity and specificity also were decreased in the pediatric population. For that reason, the authors agree with their recommendations that patients with blunt trauma with a negative POCUS examination should be followed up with additional imaging, such as computed tomography.[29]

PENETRATING TRAUMA: STAB WOUNDS

Terrorist stabbings produce injuries with a different profile and greater severity, and require more hospital resources and have worse clinical outcomes, than are seen in patients who are stabbed as a part of interpersonal conflict.[30] A detailed report from the Knife Intifada, which lasted from early 2013 to March 2016, provides data for an interesting Israeli article.[31] Patients stabbed in the setting of terrorism, for example, tended to sustain injury in the middle of the week, as opposed to victims of interpersonal violence, in whom injury was seen on the weekends. Morning and noon hours were high-risk time intervals for terror attacks, whereas the night risk was significantly higher for nonterror stabbing.[30]

Injuries sustained by patients having interpersonal conflict as opposed to patients injured by terrorism were different. Chest injuries were important in both groups but the proportion of severe chest injuries was significantly higher in the terrorism incidents. Overall volume of abdomen injuries was substantially higher after interpersonal conflict; however, severe abdominal injuries were much more common in the setting of terrorism. Patients who were stabbed in terrorist incidents had more frequent and severe injuries of the head, face, and neck. The volume of spine injuries and wounds to upper extremities resulting from terrorism by stabbing was also significantly higher. Only in the lower extremities was a similar proportion of injuries found in terrorism and interpersonal violence.[30,32,33]

Although stabbing in terrorism produced more injuries overall, patients were also more likely to arrive with unstable vital signs and a higher Revised Trauma Score and lower Glasgow Coma Score. The need for blood transfusion in patients injured by terrorism was also higher. When severity of injuries to major body regions affecting survival (head, neck, chest, and abdomen) was analyzed, among patients with injuries to those areas, the real difference between interpersonal violence and terrorist stabbing became more distinct. The likelihood of severe chest stab wounds in terrorism was 3-fold higher than with interpersonal civilian conflict. The chance of poor outcome in abdominal stab wounds was 4-fold greater in the patients injured by terrorism. Significant head injury was also more common with stabbing secondary to a terrorist event.[30,34,35]

A difference in the two patient groups was also identified from the standpoint of use of hospital resources and subsequent outcomes.[30] More than half of the patients injured by terrorism required surgery, compared with one-third of the patients who were stabbed associated with interpersonal violence. The most frequent type of surgery for patients after interpersonal civilian violence was exploratory laparotomy, whereas patients injured by terrorism required a high volume of chest and musculoskeletal procedures. The need for spine, head, eye, ear, nose, and throat procedures was also significantly higher for patients injured by terrorism. The likelihood of intensive care unit placement during hospitalization was 3-fold greater in the patients who were stabbed in association with terrorism. The requirement for imaging was also significantly higher for patients sustaining stab wounds as a part of terrorism.[30]

The general intention of terrorists is death rather than wounding or threatening. Thus, the pattern of injury commonly seen in terrorism from attacks with knives is associated with the overhand grip used to thrust downwards with the knife at a right angle to the arm. In contrast, many people injured by interpersonal violence sustain trauma from a less powerful underhand grip. Descending from the overhand position, the knife of a terrorist is most likely to strike the upper thorax, head, and neck, whereas the underhand attack in civilian conflict is directed toward the abdomen. Biomechanical studies show that the downward thrust of a terrorist assault generates greater power and knives have been shown to strike with sufficient force to penetrate bone and cartilage.[36,37] Previous Israeli studies also identify the greater length of knives used in terrorism and use of blades with greater penetrating power.[38]

WILDFIRE

Wildfire and biomass smoke exposures are increasingly recognized as an important public health issue. Although air quality in the United States has improved over the past 50 years, emissions from wildfires have trended upward and are projected to increase.[39] In 2012, wildfires in the United States contributed to 20% of all fine particulate emissions.[40] Because of projected changes secondary to drought on land cover, there is expected to be an increase in the number of wildfires in the western United States.[41,42] Wildfire smoke produces a proportionately larger amount of fine and ultrafine particulate smoke debris (defined as smaller than 2.5 and 1 μm, respectively) compared with coarse particulate matter (PM) in smoke (smaller than 10 μm).[43] These smaller particulates are a particular public health concern because they disperse farther from the source of the fire. Fire PM is noted to penetrate deeper into the airways. For this reason, PM2.5 (ie, <2.5 μm) has been singled out for special consideration in government research, tracking, and guidelines.[44]

Several studies evaluating the clinical effects of smoke inhalation from wildfires have been performed on firefighters. One of the most consistent findings is the decline in forced expiratory capacity in 1 second (FEV_1) following a season of firefighting, as found in studies by Betchley and colleagues[45] in 1997 and again by Gaughan and colleagues in 2008.[46] Swiston and colleagues[47] studied FEV_1 changes in firefighters before a shift compared with after a shift and found no significant differences, suggesting that the changes in lung function associated with PM are secondary to long-term smoke exposure and not an acute event. However, beyond physical effects, security and emotional health changes were shown in survivors of the recent wildfires in California.[48]

SUMMARY

Caused by human action or inaction, anthropogenic disasters have a differing set of clinical and social implications compared with other forms of injury (Appendix 1). For example, in the setting of blast injury, an increased pattern of severe torso injury is seen and simultaneous insults to multiple organs are found. There is a lack of extremity trauma in gunshot injuries, with head, neck, and chest injuries more often seen. As with gunshots, stab wounds in the setting of terrorism emphasize insults to the head, neck, and chest, leaving the patients with greater risk of central vascular injury. Thus, as with gunshot wounds, extremity tourniquet use in stabbings related to terrorism is less likely to be effective. In addition, as an insult of natural calamities, fires and other environmental changes leave long-term emotional and preparation issues.

REFERENCES

1. Shapira SC, Hammond JS, Cole LA. Essentials of terror medicine. New York: Springer; 2009.
2. Kapur GB, Hutson HR, Davis MA, et al. The United States twenty-year experience with bombing incidents: implications for terrorism preparedness and medical response. J Trauma 2005;59:1436–44.
3. Yeh DD, Schecter WP. Primary blast injuries—an updated concise review. World J Surg 2012;36:966–72.
4. Aharonson-Daniel L, Waisman Y, Dannon YL, et al, Members of the Israel Trauma Group. Epidemiology of terror-related versus non-terror-related traumatic injury in children. Pediatrics 2003;112(4):e280.
5. Weil YA, Peleg K, Givon A, et al. Musculoskeletal injuries in terrorist attacks - a comparison between the injuries sustained and those related to motor vehicle accidents, based on a national registry database. Injury 2008;39:1359–64.
6. Bala M, Rivkind AI, Zamir G, et al. Abdominal trauma after terrorist bombing attacks exhibits a unique pattern of injury. Ann Surg 2008;248(2):303–9.
7. Bala M, Shussman N, Rivkind AI, et al. The pattern of thoracic trauma after suicide terrorist bombing attacks. J Trauma 2010;69:1022–9.
8. Mathews ZR, Koyfman A. Blast injuries. J Emerg Med 2015;49:573–87.

9. United Nations Office on Drugs and Crime. Conventional Terrorist Weapons 2007. Available at: https://www.unodc.org/images/odccp/terrorism_weapons_conventional.html. Accessed March 11, 2019.
10. Brinsfield KH, Mitchell E Jr. The Department of Homeland Security's role in enhancing and implementing the response to active shooter and intentional mass casualty events. Bull Am Coll Surg 2015;100(Suppl):24–6.
11. Fabbri WP. The continuing threat of intentional mass casualty events in the U.S.: observations of federal law enforcement. Bull Am Coll Surg 2015;100(Suppl):47–50.
12. Smith ER, Shapiro G, Sarani B. The profile of wounding in civilian public mass shooting fatalities. J Trauma Acute Care Surg 2016;81:86–92.
13. Eastridge BJ, Mabry RL, Sequin P, et al. Death on the battlefield (2001–2011): implications for the future of combat casualty care. J Trauma Acute Care Surg 2012;73(Suppl):S431–7.
14. Champion HR, Bellamy RF, Roberts CP, et al. A profile of combat injury. J Trauma 2003;54(Suppl):S13–9.
15. Joint Committee to Create a National Policy to Enhance Survivability from Mass Casualty Shooting Events, Jacobs LM, Sinclair J, Rotondo M, et al. Active shooter and intentional mass-casualty events: the Hartford consensus II. Bull Am Coll Surg 2015;100:35–9.
16. Gregory TM, Bihel T, Guigui P, et al. Terrorist attacks in Paris: surgical trauma experience in a referral center. Injury 2016;47:2122–6.
17. Terrorist attacks by vehicle fast facts. 2017. Available at: http://www.cnn.com/2017/05/03/world/terrorist-attacks-by-vehicle-fast-facts/index.html. Accessed January 9, 2019.
18. Office of Security Policy and Industry. Engagement surface division - highway and motor carrier section. Vehicle ramming attacks: threat landscape, indicators, and countermeasures 2017; 1–7. Available at: https://publicintelligence.net/tsa-vehicle-ramming/. Accessed March 28, 2019.
19. Almogy G, Kedar A, Bala M. When a vehicle becomes a weapon: intentional vehicular assaults in Israel. Scand J Trauma Resusc Emerg Med 2016;24:149.
20. Biffl WL, Ray CE Jr, Moore EE, et al. Treatment-related outcomes from blunt cerebrovascular injuries: importance of routine follow-up arteriography. Ann Surg 2002;235:699–707.
21. Miller PR, Fabian TC, Croce MA, et al. Prospective screening for blunt cerebrovascular injuries: analysis of diagnostic modalities and outcomes. Ann Surg 2002;236:386–95.
22. Biffl WL, Moore EE, Ryu RK, et al. The unrecognized epidemic of blunt carotid arterial injuries: early diagnosis improves neurologic outcome. Ann Surg 1998;228:462–70.
23. Fabian TC, Patton JH Jr, Croce MA, et al. Blunt carotid injury. Importance of early diagnosis and anticoagulant therapy. Ann Surg 1996;223:513–25.
24. Shahan CP, Magnotti LJ, Stickley SM, et al. A safe and effective management strategy for blunt cerebrovascular injury: avoiding unnecessary anticoagulation and eliminating stroke. J Trauma Acute Care Surg 2016;80:915–22.
25. Biffl WL, Cothren CC, Moore EE, et al. Western Trauma Association critical decisions in trauma: screening for and treatment of blunt cerebrovascular injuries. J Trauma 2009;67:1150–3.
26. Scalea TM, Rodriguez A, Chiu WC, et al. Focused assessment with sonography for trauma (FAST): results from an international consensus conference. J Trauma 1999;46:466–72.

27. Alpert E, Amit U, Guranda L, et al. Emergency department point-of-care ultrasonography improves time to pericardiocentesis for clinically significant effusions. Clin Exp Emerg Med 2017;4:128–32.
28. Beck-Razi N, Fischer D, Michaelson M, et al. The utility of focused assessment with sonography for trauma as a triage tool in multiple-casualty incidents during the second Lebanon war. J Ultrasound Med 2007;26:1149–56.
29. Stengel D, Hoenning A, Leisterer J. Point-of-care ultrasonography for diagnosing thoracoabdominal injuries in patients with blunt trauma. Cochrane Database Syst Rev 2017;(9):CD012669.
30. Rozenfeld M, Givon A, Peleg K. Violence-related versus terror-related stabbings: significant differences in injury characteristics. Ann Surg 2018;267:965–70.
31. The Meir Amit Intelligence and Information Center. Initial findings of the profile of Palestinian terrorists who carried out attacks in Israel in the current wave of terrorism. 2015. Available at: http://www.terrorism-info.org.il/en/article/20900. Accessed July 7, 2016.
32. Hanoch J, Feigin E, Pikarsky A, et al. Stab wounds associated with terrorist activities in Israel. JAMA 1996;276:388–90.
33. CBS Israel. Statistical abstract of Israel. Available at: http://www.cbs.gov.il/reader/shnaton/templ_shnaton_e.html?num_tab=st04_04&CYear=2015. Accessed June 30, 2016.
34. Venara A, Jousset N, Airagnes G Jr, et al. Abdominal stab wounds: self-inflicted wounds versus assault wounds. J Forensic Leg Med 2013;20:270–3.
35. Peleg K, Jaffe DH, Israel Trauma Group. Are injuries from terror and war similar? A comparison study of civilian and soldiers. Ann Surg 2010;252:363–9.
36. Emile H, Hashmonai D. Victims of the Palestinian uprising (Intifada): a retrospective review of 220 cases. J Emerg Med 1998;16:389–94.
37. Chadwick EK, Nicol AC, Lane JV, et al. Biomechanics of knife stab attacks. Forensic Sci Int 1999;105:35–44.
38. Miller SA, Jones MD. Kinematics of four methods of stabbing: a preliminary study. Forensic Sci Int 1996;82:183–90.
39. Kinney PL. Climate change, air quality, and human health. Am J Prev Med 2008;35:459–67.
40. EPA U.S. National emissions inventory (NEI) data 2011. Available at: https://www.epa.gov/air-emissions-inventories/2011-national-emissions-inventory-nei-data. Accessed March 11, 2019.
41. Hurteau MD, Westerling AL, Wiedinmyer C, et al. Projected effects of climate and development on California wildfire emissions through 2100. Environ Sci Technol 2014;48:2298–304.
42. Abatzoglou JT, Williams AP. Impact of anthropogenic climate change on wildfire across western US forests. Proc Natl Acad Sci U S A 2016;113:11770–5.
43. Makkonen U, Hellén H, Anttila P, et al. Size distribution and chemical composition of airborne particles in south-eastern Finland during different seasons and wildfire episodes in 2006. Sci Total Environ 2010;408:644–51.
44. EPA United States Environmental Protection Agency. Integrated science assessment for particulate matter (final report) 2009. Washington, DC, Available at: https://www.epa.gov/isa/integrated-science-assessment-isa-particulate-matter. Accessed March 11, 2019.
45. Betchley C, Koenig JQ, van Belle G, et al. Pulmonary function and respiratory symptoms in forest firefighters. Am J Ind Med 1997;31:503–9.
46. Gaughan DM, Cox-Ganser JM, Enright PL, et al. Acute upper and lower respiratory effects in wildland firefighters. J Occup Environ Med 2008;50:1019–28.

47. Swiston JR, Davidson W, Attridge S, et al. Wood smoke exposure induces a pulmonary and systemic inflammatory response in firefighters. Eur Respir J 2008;32: 129–38.

48. Abbasi J. Paradise's emergency department director recalls California's worse wildfire. JAMA 2019;321:1144–6.

APPENDIX 1: AGENTS OF NATURAL AND MANMADE DISASTERS

A sample of the literature is provided in the accompanying appendix showing a variety of agents of natural and manmade disaster.[1–3] Each of the incidents is described with 1 or more references to the literature. Note that most of the articles examined did not include all required information. Thus, there is a clear need to establish a guideline for reporting on disasters.

In general, the greatest impact on population comes from natural disasters. Terrorism, for example, affects the population in more ways than simple loss of life. Response level can be described as conventional, contingency, and crisis. Conventional response uses usual patient care resources. In contingency care, patient care areas remain intact but are repurposed. A good example is the use of recovery room beds for intensive care unit–level care. When the severity of the insult requires surge response at the crisis or critical level, or facility damage does not permit usual critical care, nontraditional areas are used for critical care. More severe insults also require reorganization and acute retraining of staff, with reallocation of supplies and provision of care outside the usual clinical standards.

Location	Year	Type	Response Level	Initial Casualties	Deaths Before Admission	ER Deaths	Survivor Deaths	Admitted to Hospital	Maximum Admitted to Single Hospital	Expectant Care	Initial Transfer to OR	Initial Admission to ICU	Ventilated	Admitting Ward ICU	Admitting Ward Non-ICU
Buenos Aires[4]	1994	Bombing	—	86	2	2	5	43	86	0	6	6	NA	10	33
Tokyo[5]	1995	Nerve gas	—	651	11	1	1	111	111	0	NR	4	4	4	107
Oklahoma City[6,7]	1995	Bombing	—	759	165	3	2	83	NA	NA	25	8	10	<33	NA
Nairobi[8,9]	1998	Bombing	Critical	>5000	247	9	2	>250	250	NA	NA	NA	NA	NA	NA
New York[10-12]	2001	Airplane crash	Critical	~5000	2818	2	9	139	112	7	<23	<16	8	26	113
Singapore[13-15]	2002	SARS	Contingency	238	NR	0	33	238	238	0	NR	NA	38	45[b]	NA
Madrid[16,17]	2004	Bombing	Contingency	2062	177	9	5	509	91	NA	16	62	<83	83	426
London[18]	2005	Bombing	Contingency	775	53	0	3	NA	NA	2	12	NA	NA	7	NA
New Orleans[19]	2005	Hurricane	Critical	7508	>1800	NR	NR	~675	NA	NA	NR	NA	NA	NA	NA
Tel Aviv[20]	2006	Bombing	—	91	6	3	NA	NA	NA	3	NA	NA	NA	NA	NA
Wenchaun[21,22]	2008	Earthquake	Critical	NA	69,225	NA	NA	96,446	NA	NA	>1245[a]	NA	NA	NA	NA
Mumbai[23,24]	2008	Bombing/shooting	Contingency	476	172	NA	6	140	NA	NA	NA	NA	NA	NA	NA
Haiti[25,26]	2010	Earthquake	Critical	~500,000	~230,000	NR	NA	NR	NR	NR	>11,500[a]	NR	NA	NR	NR
East Japan[27]	2011	Earthquake/tsunami/nuclear	Critical	>25,690	15,822	NA	NA	NA	NA	NA	NA	NA	NA	NA	NA
Oslo[28,29]	2011	Bombing/shooting	Contingency/critical	227	76	0	1	43	25	0	11	21	12	32	4
San Francisco[30]	2013	Airplane crash	—	192	2	0	1	NA	19	NA	5	3	4	6	NA
Boston[31]	2013	Bombing	Contingency	281	3	0	0	75	<40	0	45	11	12	<45	19
Paris[32,33]	2015	Bombing/shooting	Contingency	382	129	2	2	302	53	NA	76	NA	NA	42	NA
Brussels[34]	2016	Bombing	—	375	35	NA	NA	NA	NA	NA	NA	NA	NA	NA	NA
Nice[35,36]	2016	Truck ramming	Contingency	456	76	8	2	98	NA	NA	18	8	NA	20	78
Las Vegas[37,38]	2017	Shooting	Contingency	927	31	26	1	185	75	NA	NA	NA	NA	63	122

Some data are approximate because various sources provide disparate data.

Abbreviations: NA, not available; NR, not reported; SARS, severe acute respiratory syndrome.

[a] Including all surgery.

[b] At any point during hospitalization.

REFERENCES

1. Christian MD, Devereaux AV, Dichter JR, et al. Introduction and executive summary: care of the critically ill and injured during pandemics and disasters: CHEST consensus statement. Chest 2014;146(Suppl):8S–34S.
2. Hick JL, Barbera JA, Kelen GD. Refining surge capacity: conventional, contingency, and crisis capacity. Disaster Med Public Health Prep 2009;3(Suppl): S59–67.
3. Ornelas J, Dichter JR, Devereaux AV, et al. Methodology: care of the critically ill and injured during pandemics and disasters: CHEST consensus statement. Chest 2014;146(Suppl):35S–41S.
4. Biancolini CA, Del Bosco CG, Jorge MA. Argentine Jewish community institution bomb explosion. J Trauma 1999;47(4):728–32.
5. Okumura T, Takasu N, Ishimatsu S, et al. Report on 640 victims of the Tokyo subway sarin attack. Ann Emerg Med 1996;28(2):129–35.
6. Mallonee S, Shariat S, Stennies G, et al. Physical injuries and fatalities resulting from the Oklahoma City Bombing. JAMA 1996;276(5):382–7.
7. Hogan DE, Waeckerle JF, Dire DJ, et al. Emergency department impact of the Oklahoma city terrorist bombing. Ann Emerg Med 1999;34(2):160–7.
8. Kalebi A, Olumbe A. Forensic findings from the Nairobi U.S. embassy terrorist bombing. East Afr Med J 2006;83(7):380–8.
9. Abdallah S, Heinzen R, Burnham G. Immediate and long-term assistance following the bombing of the US Embassies in Kenya and Tanzania. Disasters 2007;31(4):417–34.
10. Cushman JG, Pachter HL, Beaton HL. Two New York City hospitals' surgical response to the September 11, 2001, terrorist attack in New York City. J Trauma 2003;54(1):147–54 [discussion: 154–5].
11. Pryor JP. The 2001 world trade center disaster: summary and evaluation of experiences. Eur J Trauma Emerg Surg 2009;35:212–36.
12. Kirschenbaum L, Keene A, O'Neill P, et al. The experience at St. Vincent's Hospital, Manhattan, on September 11, 2001: preparedness, response, and lessons learned. Crit Care Med 2005;33(Supplement):S48–52.
13. Goh K-T, Cutter J, Heng B-H, et al. Epidemiology and control of SARS in Singapore. Ann Acad Med Singapore 2006;35(5):301–16.
14. Gopalakrishna G, Choo P, Leo YS, et al. SARS transmission and hospital containment. Emerg Infect Dis 2004;10(3):395–400.
15. Chong PY, Chui P, Ling AE, et al. Analysis of deaths during the severe acute respiratory syndrome (SARS) epidemic in Singapore: challenges in determining a SARS diagnosis. Arch Pathol Lab Med 2004;128(2):195–204.
16. Turégano-Fuentes F, Caba-Doussoux P, Jover-Navalón JM, et al. Injury patterns from major urban terrorist bombings in trains: the Madrid experience. World J Surg 2008;32(6):1168–75.
17. Turégano-Fuentes F, Pérez-Díaz D, Sanz-Sánchez M, et al. Overall asessment of the response to terrorist bombings in trains, Madrid, 11 March 2004. Eur J Trauma Emerg Surg 2008;34(5):433–41.
18. Aylwin CJ, König TC, Brennan NW, et al. Reduction in critical mortality in urban mass casualty incidents: analysis of triage, surge, and resource use after the London bombings on July 7, 2005. Lancet 2006;368(9554):2219–25.
19. Stratton SJ, Tyler RD. Characteristics of medical surge capacity demand for sudden-impact disasters. Acad Emerg Med 2006;13:1193–7.

20. Raiter Y, Farfel A, Lehavi O, et al. Mass casualty incident management, triage, injury distribution of casualties and rate of arrival of casualties at the hospitals: lessons from a suicide bomber attack in downtown Tel Aviv. Emerg Med J 2008;25(4):225–9.

21. Lu-Ping Z, Rodriguez-Llanes JM, Qi W, et al. Multiple injuries after earthquakes: a retrospective analysis on 1871 injured patients from the 2008 Wenchuan earthquake. Crit Care 2012;16(3):R87.

22. Qiu J, Liu G, Wang S, et al. Analysis of injuries and treatment of 3 401 inpatients in 2008 Wenchuan earthquake—based on Chinese Trauma databank. Chin J Traumatol 2010;13(5):297–303.

23. Bhandarwar AH, Bakhshi GD, Tayade MB, et al. Surgical response to the 2008 Mumbai terror attack. Br J Surg 2012;99(3):368–72.

24. Roy N, Kapil V, Subbarao I, et al. Mass casualty response in the 2008 Mumbai terrorist attacks. Disaster Med Public Health Prep 2011;5(04):273–9.

25. McIntyre T, Hughes CD, Pauyo T, et al. Emergency surgical care delivery in post-earthquake Haiti: partners in health and Zanmi Lasante experience. World J Surg 2011;35(4):745–50.

26. Gerdin M, Wladis A, von Schreeb J. Foreign field hospitals after the 2010 Haiti earthquake: how good were we? Emerg Med J 2013;30(1):e8.

27. Ishii M, Nagata T. The Japan Medical Association's disaster preparedness: lessons from the Great East Japan earthquake and Tsunami. Disaster Med Public Health Prep 2013;7(05):507–12.

28. Waage S, Poole JC, Thorgersen EB. Rural hospital mass casualty response to a terrorist shooting spree. Br J Surg 2013;100(9):1198–204.

29. Gaarder C, Jorgensen J, Kolstadbraaten KM, et al. The twin terrorist attacks in Norway on July 22, 2011. J Trauma Acute Care Surg 2012;73(1):269–75.

30. Campion EM, Juillard C, Knudson MM, et al. Reconsidering the resources needed for multiple casualty events. JAMA Surg 2016;151(6):512.

31. Gates JD, Arabian S, Biddinger P, et al. The initial response to the Boston marathon bombing: lessons learned to prepare for the next disaster. Ann Surg 2014; 260(6):960–6.

32. Hirsch M, Carli P, Nizard R, et al. The medical response to multisite terrorist attacks in Paris. Lancet 2015;386(10012):2535–8.

33. Philippe J-M, Brahic O, Carli P, et al. French Ministry of Health's response to Paris attacks of 13 November 2015. Crit Care 2016;20(1):85.

34. Compernolle V, Najdovski T, De Bouyalski I, et al. Lessons for blood services following the Brussels terrorist attacks in March 2016. ISBT Sci Ser 2018;13(1): 47–50.

35. Orban J-C, Quintard H, Ichai C. ICU specialists facing terrorist attack: the Nice experience. Intensive Care Med 2017;43(5):683–5.

36. Massalou D, Ichai C, Mariage D, et al. Terrorist attack in Nice – the experience of general surgeons. J Visc Surg 2019;156(1):17–22.

37. Lozada MJ, Cai S, Li M, et al. The Las Vegas mass shooting. J Trauma Acute Care Surg 2019;86(1):128–33.

38. Kuhls DA, Fildes JJ, Johnson M, et al. Southern Nevada trauma system uses proven techniques to save lives after 1 October shooting. Bull Am Coll Surg 2018;103(3):39–45.

Provision of Care for Critically Ill Children in Disasters

Mitchell Hamele, MD[a],*, Ramon E. Gist, MD[b], Niranjan Kissoon, MD[c]

KEYWORDS

- Disaster • Pediatrics • Mass critical care • Children • Critical illness • Injuries
- Trauma

KEY POINTS

- Children are disproportionately affected in disasters.
- The current state of pediatric disaster preparedness, although improving, is suboptimal and deserves attention across all jurisdictions.
- Children have unique vulnerabilities and needs that must be addressed in disaster planning and provision of care.

INTRODUCTION

Children are disproportionately affected in all types of disasters including natural, infectious, and conflict related.[1,2] Children are more vulnerable compared with adults because of physiologic, anatomic, and psychosocial differences. Despite this, planning at the national, local, and health care facility levels tends to focus on adults.[3] This oversight poses significant risks to the 69 million children younger than age 18 in the United States, which represents nearly one-quarter of the population.[4]

Often routine pediatric emergency care is suboptimal because many receive care at hospitals with inadequate pediatric-trained personnel and pediatric-specific equipment.[5] In 2010 the National Commission on Children and Disasters delivered a comprehensive report with specific recommendations to the US government

Disclosure Statement: LTC M. Hamele is an officer in the United States Army. The views in this article are those of the authors and do not reflect the views of the United States Army, Department of Defense, or the United States Government.

[a] Department of Pediatrics-Critical Care, Tripler Army Medical Center, Honolulu, HI 96859, USA; [b] Department of Pediatrics, Division of Pediatric Critical Care Medicine, SUNY Downstate Medical Center, 450 Clarkson Avenue, Box 49, Brooklyn, NY 11203, USA; [c] Department of Pediatrics and Emergency Medicine, BC Children's Hospital, Sunny Hill Health Centre for Children, UBC, Child and Family Research Institute, B245 - 4480 Oak Street, Vancouver, British Columbia V6H 3V4, Canada
* Corresponding author.
E-mail addresses: mitchell.t.hamele.mil@mail.mil; mthamele@yahoo.com

designed to close an alarming number of gaps in pediatric all-hazards disaster preparedness.[6] This report and subsequent legislation has largely been ignored as illustrated by a 2015 report by Save the Children, which found less than 0.1% of federal emergency preparedness funds are directed toward activities targeting children and 79% of the National Commission's recommendations remained unfulfilled.[7] Only 6% of emergency departments have the recommended pediatric equipment,[8] only half of Children's Hospital Association members are certified in the National Disaster Medical System, and hospital disaster funding is limited and highly variable.[9]

These planning gaps increase the likelihood that a disaster will have a greater negative impact on children when compared with adults. New voluntary regional coalitions have been developed to fill this gap. Some are pediatric focused (Mountain States Pediatric Disaster Coalition) or have pediatrics well integrated into the greater coalition (Northwest Healthcare Response Network) (**Table 1**). Whether sheltering in place, ensuring safe evacuations, or accepting surges of patients, the pediatric intensive care unit (PICU) plays a central role in disaster responses. It is essential for PICU and adult ICU practitioners to understand their role in the framework of a larger disaster response and how the approach to patient care changes under these conditions. The objectives of this review are to highlight some of these specifics, which include:

- Essentials of formulating a pediatric disaster plan
- Special clinical considerations
- Ethical issues

ESSENTIALS OF FORMULATING A PEDIATRIC DISASTER PLAN

Formulating a pediatric disaster plan involves attention to the following elements: crisis standards of care (CSC), triage, stuff, staff, space, and systems.

Crisis Standards of Care

The institutional readiness and ability to deploy CSC are integral in preparation to provide care for children in any disaster. CSC is defined by the Institute of Medicine

Table 1
Selected pediatric disaster planning resources and agencies

Name	Web site
American Academy of Pediatrics: Children & Disasters	https://www.aap.org/en-us/advocacy-and-policy/aap-health-initiatives/Children-and-Disasters/Pages/default.aspx
Centers for Disease Control and Prevention: Caring for Children in a Disaster	https://www.cdc.gov/childrenindisasters/index.html
HHS-Agency for Healthcare Research and Quality: Public Health Emergency and Preparedness	https://disaster.nlm.nih.gov/dimrc/children.html
HHS-Office of the Assistant Secretary for Preparedness and Response	https://www.phe.gov/about/pages/default.aspx
Mountain States Pediatric Disaster Coalition	http://mspdc.org/
Northwest Healthcare Response Network	https://nwhrn.org/
World Health Organization: Emergencies Preparedness, Response	http://www.who.int/csr/en/

as "a substantial change in usual health care operations and the level of care it is possible to deliver, which is made necessary by a pervasive (eg, pandemic influenza) or catastrophic (eg, earthquake, hurricane) disaster."[10] These altered standards must include legal and regulatory protection for institutions and staff who may need to provide care for children outside of their normal scope of practice.[11] Although ideally this declaration would come from a public agency, when planning it is important for institutions to codify their own triggers and standards for their institutional CSC.

Triage and Children

Triage is an important component of provision of care for children in disasters. Triage serves two purposes: to sort patients to appropriate locations, which requires regional coordination; and to ensure optimal use of limited resources. Children are often transported or present at the closest facility regardless of capabilities to provide care, emphasizing the need for a regionalized triage system.[12] Primary (sorting by priority at the scene) and secondary triage (priority and disposition at a treatment facility) systems should dictate pediatric patient flow if regional pediatric triage plans are in place.[13] PICU directors and other pediatric specialists (eg, surgeons) are responsible for tertiary triage decisions related to the priority and definitive management of critically ill patients, but should also be involved in development and adoption of regional primary and secondary pediatric triage systems.

Despite the importance of triage to allocate resource usage during a disaster there are no pediatric triage systems that are effective or validated.[13] While developing pediatric triage systems the likelihood of survival and the need for extended resource use should be considered and the triage system should be population based and system wide.[13] A retrospective pediatric model using this approach with CSC implementation demonstrated improved population survival.[14] A pediatric triage system that allocates patients across pediatric and adult facilities would be most effective in a large-scale disaster.[13,15] Pediatric triage systems should also consider the unique vulnerabilities of children; the inability to avoid dangerous exposures, increased minute ventilation, susceptibility to hypothermia, inability to independently care for themselves or present for care, and need for identification and family reunification.[3,16] While developing a local or regional system it is important to involve a multidisciplinary team including neonatal ICUs, emergency medical services, adult/community hospitals, schools, and governmental agencies.[17]

Stuff

Stuff refers to the supplies needed to provide care for children in a disaster. Most hospitals retain only enough supplies to sustain 3 to 5 days of normal operations. This just-in-time supply system is insufficient during disasters when facilities providing pediatric critical care may be called on to provide from 200% to 300% of peak capacity for up to 10 to 42 days.[18] Several committees and institutions have developed standardized pediatric supply lists including one with recommendations for a 10-bed PICU.[18,19] Just-in-time supply chains need to be supplemented by access to regional stockpiles with interoperable and compatible supplies, facility-based caches of pediatric supplies, supplies that can be reused or cross-leveled (eg, using 1-L bags for infants and children or cuffed endotracheal tubes only), dual sourcing of high-priority nonsubstitutable items, and an integrated tracking system.[18,20] Additionally planners should consider that the age distribution in a disaster will include more school and adolescent patients than is typical in normal operations in which young children predominate.[18]

The ability to provide mechanical ventilator support is the factor that determines the capability to provide intensive care support. However, less than half of stockpiled ventilators in the United States possess the minimum alarm functionality and ability to deliver safe tidal volumes in infants.[21] During the H1N1 outbreak proportionally more children required mechanical ventilation than adults and mortality increased significantly in a setting of limited ventilator availability.[22,23] It is important to consider alternate modes of delivery of mechanical ventilation during disasters, such as use of patients' home ventilators, transport ventilators, anesthesia ventilators in the PICU, triaged distribution of neonatal ICU ventilators, and noninvasive positive pressure ventilators.[18] The ability to provide ventilator support should be incorporated in the institutional and regional CSC because ventilator triage carries significant ethical and medical-legal ramifications.

Medications in pediatric-appropriate delivery systems and appropriately sized equipment is another important consideration that is poorly served by national stockpiles.[3] Focus on pediatric formulations of medications with broad application for stockpiling is most cost effective. Examples include crystalloids, vasopressors, broad-spectrum antimicrobials, sedative and analgesic medications, and enteral nutrition.[13,18] Extending medication shelf-life and restricted usage of an emergency stockpile can also increase supply.[13]

Plans for care of children should also include incubators, radiant warmers, or the means to environmentally heat patient care areas because children are at high risk of hypothermia.[18] CSC should also include how, when, and whether to allocate advanced life support modalities, such as dialysis or extracorporeal life support, which have been shown to improve outcomes in disaster but may be too resource intensive in many health care settings.[24,25] Pediatric critical care disaster planners should also consider the supplies needed to care for the families of their patients and personal protective equipment stockpiles.

Staff

During a disaster up to 60% of staff may be unavailable for work.[26] Illness, fatigue, fear, infrastructure damage, and caregiver duties would all limit staff availability.[27] To mitigate staff shortages hospitals should provide for the rest, shelter, nutrition, and transportation needs of staff and their families.[28] Staff training on infection control procedures, rigorous vaccination, and staff health monitoring plans all limit staff loss because of illness.

Pediatric critical care physicians are a significant limiting factor with less than 2000 board-certified pediatric intensivists in the United States with variable state-to-state density.[29] Regional strategies to augment physician shortages and to maximize care capabilities at nonpediatric hospitals could include: use of emergency credentialing of adult providers to care for postpubertal pediatric patients, local or telephonic expert consultation to assist nonpediatric critical care trained providers, movement of skilled pediatric critical care teams to nonpediatric centers, extended work hours, repatriation of trainees, and elimination of educational rounds.[11,27]

Attention to the nonphysician team should include planning for nursing and other specialty professional care. Health care chaplains, palliative care experts, and parents should be involved in planning and care of children and may augment nursing care.[13] Nursing plans should include cross-training on a regular basis, "just-in-time" training, use of pediatric surgical and emergency staff, blended care teams (eg, two pediatric critical care nurses supervising three ward nurses with seven patients), altered staff to patient ratios, and tracking staff at primarily adult hospitals with pediatric training.[13,18,28] Training in disaster medicine should be included in orientation and annual training.[30] When developing institutional CSC it is vital to include medical-legal protections for staff operating outside their typical scope or practice parameters.[11,31]

Space

In the United States there are 4 to 5000 PICU beds and 80,000 adult ICU beds.[32,33] A quarter of the US population is younger than 18 years old and disasters tend to disproportionally effect children. With 5% of the existing bed capacity and greater than 20% of the population space to provide pediatric critical care will be a significant challenge in national or regional disasters and may be exacerbated by structural damage if existing PICUs are damaged.[2,34] At children's hospitals care could be provided in nonstandard monitored locations, such as postanesthesia recovery units, operating rooms (OR), and other procedural areas with monitoring capability.[13,28,31] Elective procedures should be canceled and discharge or transfer criteria should be lowered.[28,31] These decisions should be included in institutional CSC and consider the type of disaster because earthquakes or hurricanes may require increased surgical care in the first few days followed by increased medical care needs, unlike pandemics during which OR resources could initially be shunted to primarily medical care.[35]

At adult hospitals tele-health or regional pediatric specialty team support of pediatric patients in monitored areas (ICU, post anesthesia care unit [PACU], OR, emergency department) may maximize space and is contingent on multidisciplinary regional organization.[13,27] These facilities could also be used as "satellite" units to care for critically ill pediatric patients not directly related to the disaster or to cohort noninfectious patients and staff in pandemics.[27] Technology-dependent pediatric patients only in need of emergency power could be diverted to adult facilities with families providing care using medical equipment brought from home.

Space for storage and removal of waste (infectious and noninfectious) should be included in planning.[36] Consideration should be given to locations and facilities to shelter and feed families of ill patients, staff members, and potentially families of staff members.[37] Adequate space for safe, respectful care of the deceased, away from patient care areas should also be addressed when looking at systems and space.[38]

Systems

A multidisciplinary team and coordinated system must be in place to implement and coordinate any of the previously mentioned recommendations to provide pediatric critical care in a disaster. A team comprised of local government services, community leaders, pharmacy support, nutritional services, security personnel, school officials, and pediatric physicians, nurses, other clinical leaders and health care administrators must be engaged in the planning phase of disaster response. A clear command structure, local and regional, with clearly defined roles and lines of communication should be defined and enshrined in protocols and procedures once the rules and processes by which critically ill pediatric patients should be allocated are established.[13,31] The command structure should have the ability to coordinate expansion or restriction of pediatric critical care resources, facilitate the flow of critical equipment, patients, and specialty pediatric teams to nonpediatric facilities and implement CSC regionally. These processes should be trialed regularly in local and regional "tabletop" exercises in a multidisciplinary manner. Existing pediatric trauma centers may be well suited to facilitate this role.[39]

A clearly articulated and robust system for identifying and tracking children during disasters is important. Its importance was underlined during Katrina when more than 2700 children were initially missing with only 26% located after 2 weeks.[40] A working group of the Pediatric Disaster Resource and Training Center with the US Department of Health and Human Services published 48 wide-ranging recommendations for family reunification.[41] Keys to implementation are advanced planning for communication throughout the regional system of care; inclusion of law enforcement, transport services, schools and daycare centers in planning; and pre-designation of appropriate transport teams and triage criteria for pediatric-specific versus community hospitals with a multidisciplinary tracking system.[3,20,37,42,43] Proto-cols designed for waiver of consent, photographic tracking within the system, and regional distribution of pediatric patients should be nested within local and regional CSC.[3,37,42,43] The National Center for Missing and Exploited Children Unaccompanied Minor Registry is another reunification resource available at: https://umr.missingkids.org/umr/reportUMR?execution=e1s1.

Reliable and trusted communication systems should also be determined and tested for rapid distribution of clinical and logistic information among medical trans-port teams, hospitals, and the community at large.[13,38,43] The system to communi-cate must be trusted and consistent.[38] Communication of educational materials should consider potential disruptions to infrastructure-dependent systems and include targeted clinical just-in-time training and more comprehensive advanced training (**Table 2**) for personnel who typically care for adults but may need to care for children in a disaster.[44] Security personnel and protocols should be considered given the high degree of stress, dislocation, and resource limitation in a large-scale disaster. Finally, effective communication in a disaster is dependent on existing community involvement and relationships that are developed during regular exer-cises that stress regional pediatric disaster plans. Overview of pediatric-specific planning is shown in **Table 3**.

SPECIAL CLINICAL CONSIDERATIONS

Educating health care providers on the clinically relevant differences between children and adults is important in disaster planning and execution. Pediatricians who regularly care for children and adult providers may be unfamiliar with the nuances of caring for children in disasters.[45] The interdependent characteristics that make children uniquely susceptible to harm during a disaster fall into four categories: (1) anatomic, (2) phys-iologic, (3) developmental, and (4) psychological.[46]

Table 2 Advanced comprehensive training products for pediatric disaster		
	Focus	Resource Sites
Pediatric Advanced Life Support (American Heart Association)	Improve the quality and care provided to seriously ill children	https://international.heart.org/en/our-courses/pediatric-advanced-life-support
Pediatric Fundamentals of Critical Care Support	Recognition of critical illness and initiation of care for the critically ill pediatric patient in the absence of an intensivist	http://www.sccm.org/Fundamentals/Pediatric-Fundamental-Critical-Care-Support
TEEX Pediatric Disaster Response and Emergency Preparedness	Prepares students to plan for and respond to a disaster incident involving children, in the event of a community based-incident	https://teex.org/Pages/Class.aspx?course=MGT439&courseTitle=Pediatric+Disaster+Response+and+Emergency+Preparedness

Table 3
Pediatric disaster planning: stuff, staff, space, systems

Area of Planning	Threats	Mitigation Strategies
Stuff: the supplies needed to provide care and support for patients, staff, and families	1. Need to operate at 2%–300% of normal volume for 10 d 2. Limited supplies of critical equipment/ medication 3. Limited supplies of support material (food, water, personal protective equipment)	1. CSC and established triage and treatment protocols (restricted medication usage, extended shelf lives) 2. (a) Local/regional stockpiles of interoperable/ compatible supplies; and (b) advocacy for governmental planning for pediatric contingencies 3. Multidisciplinary planning team; realistic estimate of support needs including patient attendants, staff, and their families
Staff: the trained personnel needed to care for patients, their families, and other staff	1. 10%–60% absenteeism 2. Increased need for pediatric critical care staff beyond available assets	1. (a) Plan for housing, feeding, and transporting staff and their families; (b) aggressive staff vaccination of infection control policies; and (c) altered staffing with blended "care teams" and extended hours 2. (a) Emergency credentials with consultation and mobile specialty pediatric teams at adult facilities; and (b) advanced pediatric and "just-in-time training" programs for adult and pediatric staff

(continued on next page)

Table 3
(continued)

Area of Planning	Threats	Mitigation Strategies
Space: appropriate physical areas to provide patient care and support services	1. Limited existing bed space for pediatric critical care 2. Limited space for support services (eg, waste, deceased, nutrition) 3. Limited space for family members (patients and staff)	1. (a) Adoption of crisis standards of care; canceling of "elective" procedures; (b) using adult spaces for pediatric critical care; and (c) use of all monitored areas for critical care (eg, PACU, OR, ED) 2. Coordination with local support and government services 3. Planning for mobile or temporary "camps"
Systems: the coordinate command and control centers that provide efficient, coordinated flow of resources, patients, and information	1. Need for interfacility communication/coordination 2. Need to track patients 3. Need to standardize standards of care and triage 4. Need to provide safe care environment	1. Establishment of regional and local command centers with lines of communication with pediatric expertise 2. Develop regional system of patient tracking and information sharing 3. Establish local/regional/national CSC for pandemics and large-scale disasters with standardized educational products 4. Involve local law enforcement and security services in planning

Abbreviation: ED, emergency department.

Anatomy

The ratio of surface area to body weight is larger in children than adults. Infants and toddlers also have a thinner epidermis with increased perfusion.[47] When exposed to a skin-permeable toxin, a child can absorb a high dose and soap and warm water is preferred for decontamination because typical decontamination agents are caustic to them.[47,48] Children are prone to develop hypothermia when exposed to the elements or when undergoing decontamination.[46] The high surface area to mass ratio increases the risk for severe injuries and increased fluid losses from burn injuries.

Children are more vulnerable to solid organ damage resulting from blunt trauma and blast waves.[48] They are smaller in mass, with less adipose and connective tissue than adults. Compliant bones enable transmission of energy to underlying organs and the ribs do not protect their large liver and spleen from blunt trauma.

A child's airway is significantly different from that of an adult. The tongue is large for the mouth, the epiglottis is large and floppy, the larynx is anterior and superior, the airway is narrowest at the cricoid cartilage, and the trachea is narrow and compliant. Because of this smaller children are susceptible to obstruction and dynamic collapse and the anatomy of the pediatric airway makes endotracheal intubation challenging. Children are also at risk for inhaling various toxins at higher doses because of their disproportionately increased minute ventilation.[46]

Children have proportionately larger heads and a short neck with underdeveloped muscle strength supporting the head and cervical spine and thin cranial bones putting them at risk for severe injuries from head and neck trauma. As a child grows, the brain undergoes a myriad of changes that leads to further cognitive and social development and neuronal injury can result in permanent injury and developmental arrest.

Physiology

Circulating blood volume relative to weight decreases with age (neonates, 85–90 mL/kg; infant, 80–85 mL/kg; children, 70–75 mL/kg; adults, 65–70 mL/kg); however, the absolute blood volume in small children is low.[49] Children have immature nephrons that are unable to effectively conserve water. Unlike adults, children can mount a strong compensatory response to shock via tachycardia and systemic vasoconstriction. These factors make early recognition of volume loss and shock difficult in children. Hypotension is a late sign indicating that a child is in uncompensated shock and at high risk for developing cardiopulmonary arrest.[46]

Development and Psychology

The developmental milestones a child has achieved when disaster occurs impacts their ability to survive and cope. Infants and toddlers are not developmentally self-sufficient and may exhibit separation and stranger anxiety. A variety of psychological sequelae are possible after a disaster, which are affected by chronologic and developmental ages. Younger children are unable to escape danger or follow directions during an evacuation. Children may react negatively to rescuers or care providers wearing fear-provoking personal protective equipment. Separating children from family members should be avoided as much as possible. Medical staff need to be prepared to manage a myriad of psychological responses during the acute and recovery phases from a disaster.[46,50]

Natural Disasters

Natural disasters have been a consistent threat to life and infrastructure throughout American history. Floods, earthquakes, hurricanes, tornados, and fires are the most common types of disasters. These events impact children differently than adults. Infants and toddlers are unable to escape danger without the help of caregivers, which increases the likelihood of them experiencing physical harm. The health care infrastructure can be compromised, making it difficult for injured children to access care. This is particularly concerning for children with special needs who are dependent on medical technology.[51]

The long-term effects of natural disasters are equally devastating. Loss of shelter, inadequate nutrition, and unsanitary conditions are common after a natural disaster and disproportionly effect children. Contamination of the water supply can lead to infectious disease outbreaks, such as diarrheal illnesses that impact younger children greatly because of their deficient fluid reserves. Natural disasters also have lasting effects on a child's mental health. As an example, children who lived through Hurricane Katrina experienced an increased incidence of post-traumatic stress disorder. It is difficult for a child to cope if a parent/guardian is missing, injured, or killed. Finally, interruptions in a young child's schooling can cause long-term developmental impairments.[51]

CHEMICAL, BIOLOGIC, RADIATION, NUCLEAR, AND EXPLOSIVE DISASTERS

Children are at higher risk for injury and death from disasters involving chemical, biologic, radiation, nuclear, and explosive disasters hazards because of their inherent vulnerabilities. In contrast to natural disasters, most of these events are anthropogenic. Exposure to these hazards can occur because of human error; however, terrorism must be considered as a potential cause when any of these hazards are involved.[48]

Chemicals

Disasters involving chemical hazards typically occur in the setting of an industrial accident or terrorist attack. Chemicals are placed into categories based on the organ systems they target: respiratory, mucocutaneous, lacrimatory, and neurologic.[48] Cyanogens are another important class.[52] Symptoms in children are the same as adults with all agents with the following additional vulnerabilities and treatment considerations (**Table 4**).

Table 4		
Pediatric dosing for management of chemical agents		
Agent	**Pediatric Dosage**	**Notes**
Nerve agents	Atropine 0.5 mg/kg IV or IM q 2–5 min (max 5 mg)	Repeat for recurrent symptoms
	Pralidoxime 25 mg/kg IV or IM q 1 h (max 1 g IV or 2 g IM)	May use Mark I kits for children >2 y: 3–7 y (1 kit max) 8–14 y (2 kit max) >14 y (3 kit max)
Seizure treatment	Midazolam IM 0.2 mg/kg (max 10 mg) *OR* Lorazepam IV/IM 0.1 mg/kg (max 4 mg)	Repeat q 5 min as needed × 2
Cyanide	Hydroxocobalamin 70 mg/kg (max 5 g), first-line *OR* Sodium nitrate 0.33 mL/kg IV followed by sodium thiosulfate (25%) 1.65 mL/kg IV (max 50 mL)	May repeat hydroxocobalamin × 1 as needed

Abbreviations: IM, intramuscularly; IV, intravenously.

- Chlorine and phosgene are dense gases that settle near the ground and are inhaled at high doses by children because of their proximity to the ground and higher minute ventilation.[46,48] Decontamination with warm soap and water and airway management are the mainstays of treatment in children.
- Children are at increased risk of rapid absorption of mucocutaneous agents and rapid decontamination with warm soap and water is critical to prevent further absorption is critical.
- Organophosphates are neurologic agents used in farming as pesticides and in terrorism as nerve agents: tabun, sarin, soman, VX, and novichok, which was used in a targeted attack in the United Kingdom.[53] Children are at greater risk of accidental exposure to farming pesticides in the disaster setting. Decontamination and resuscitation are initial priorities.

Cyanide salts and sodium azide are cyanogens; children more vulnerable because of higher metabolic activity of the brain and heart. Decontamination is not typically indicated.[54] Cyanide antidote kits can cause nitrate-induced hypotension and methemoglobinemia, particularly in children. Hydroxocobalamin is now the first-line therapy.[16]

In children decontamination is complicated by hypothermia and skin injury. Excessive secretions or debris increases the intrinsic risk for airway obstruction. Many of these chemicals cause bronchospasm, which tends to be more severe in children and should be managed with β_2-agonists and corticosteroids. Goal-directed fluid resuscitation is essential because losses may be underestimated, whereas excessive fluid resuscitation can exacerbate lung injury.[48]

Biologics

Disasters involving biologic hazards can occur through human-to-human transmission, zoonotic transmission, or terrorism. The Centers for Disease Control and Prevention groups biologics into categories A, B, and C. Category A agents are the most dangerous of these and pediatric considerations are discussed next.[16,48] Where not noted the pathophysiology and symptoms are similar to adults. Antimicrobial treatment, when indicated, is outlined in **Table 5**.

- Smallpox was declared eradicated by the World Health Organization in 1980 and terrorism should be suspected with any new cases.[55] Infected patients should be placed on contact and airborne isolation precautions. Close contacts, including children, should receive the smallpox vaccine within 3 to 4 days of exposure.[48]
- *Bacillus anthracis* symptoms and mortality in children are similar to adults. No isolation precautions are indicated, because person-to-person spread has not been documented.[16]
- *Clostridium botulinum* causes descending paralysis leading to respiratory failure and death once the diaphragm is affected. Infantile botulism is naturally occurring, sporadic, and may increase in disasters because of aerosolized spores in soil. Treatment involves supportive measures including mechanical ventilation, total parenteral nutrition, and administration of antitoxin to halt progression of disease.
- *Yersinia pestis* causes plague and if weaponized and inhaled manifests as sepsis, disseminated intravascular coagulopathy, and death if untreated.[48] Patients should be placed on contact and droplet isolation and close contacts should receive exposure prophylaxis.[54]
- Tularemia is caused by *Francisella tularensis* and aerosol dissemination during a terrorist attack leads to pleuropneumonitis.[48] No isolation-specific precautions are indicated.[54]

Table 5
Pediatric management of biologic agents

Agent	Pediatric Dose	Notes
Inhalational anthrax	Ciprofloxacin 10–15 mg/kg (max 400 mg) IV q 12 h OR Doxycycline 2.2 mg/kg (max 100 mg) IV q 12 h PLUS clindamycin 10–15 mg/kg q 8 h OR Penicillin G 400–600 U/kg/d IV divided q 4 h	Switch to oral therapy when patient shows signs of improvement. At least one agent should have good CNS penetration.
	Prophylaxis for exposed: Ciprofloxacin 15 mg/kg po q 12 h OR Doxycycline 2.2 mg/kg IV q 12 h	Prophylaxis is for a 60-d course.
Plague or tularemia (treatment is the same for both)	Gentamycin 2.5 mg/kg IV q 8 h OR Streptomycin 15 mg/kg IM q 12 h (max 2 mg/d) OR Doxycycline 2.2 mg/kg IV q 12 h (max 200 mg/d) OR Ciprofloxacin 15 mg/kg IV q 12 h	
	Prophylaxis for exposed: trimethoprim/sulfa 4 mg/kg po q 12 h	Prophylaxis is for a 5–7 d course.
Botulism	Infants <1 y human-derived botulinum immunoglobulin "Baby BIG" Children >1 y equine serum botulism antitoxin	In United States call 1-800-222-1222 or 770-488-7100. Outside United States contact local health agencies.

Abbreviations: CNS, central nervous system; IM, intramuscularly; IV, intravenously.

- Viral hemorrhagic fever (VHF) is caused by a myriad of RNA viruses including the Ebola virus.[48] The Ebola outbreak of 2014 demonstrated that person-to-person transmission of VHF continues to pose a significant threat.[56–58] VHF symptoms and treatment in children are similar as in adults and largely supportive. Decontamination of patient care areas and equipment with hypochlorite or phenolic agents is critical.[48]

Radiologic and Nuclear

Growing children have rapidly dividing cells that are susceptible to damage from ionizing radiation, which can lead to secondary malignancies. The eyes of children are also sensitive to radiation damage. Their thinner skin and large surface area relative to weight increases the chance of causing severe burn injury and absorbing a higher radiation dose absorbed than adults.[54] Higher minute ventilation rates and proximity to the ground increases their risk for inhalational contamination, whereas their propensity for pica creates a higher risk for enteral contamination.[48] Toxicity through ingestion is also a concern because cow milk and human milk can be contaminated during radiologic disasters.[59] Adult bioassays are used to determine the internalized dose of radiation in children because there is limited knowledge on pediatric biologic dosimetry.[48] Long-term follow-up is needed to monitor for psychological and oncologic sequelae. Children are 10 times as likely to develop a thyroid malignancy than an adult exposed to the same radiation dose. As such, pregnant or lactating women, and children of all ages who are exposed should receive prophylaxis with potassium iodide.[48]

Explosive

In 2017, blast events involving various forms of explosive devices were the most common type of terrorist event.[59] Blast injuries are challenging because they combine conventional trauma injuries with the unique impact of blast waves, whose effects are more devastating for children.[48] The subsequent societal fear and various psychological sequelae are long lasting.[60]

Blast lung and gastrointestinal injuries may be difficult to detect in children because of poor communication but manifest similarly as adults with dyspnea, hemoptysis, and abdominal injuries. Blast auditory injury may be difficult to detect in traumatized children without use of an otoscope but if discovered they are discharged after 6 hours with otolaryngology follow-up if they are otherwise asymptomatic and have a normal chest radiograph.[60]

Young children have increased vagal tone and are at high risk for blast-related hypotension and bradycardia. This can lead to excessive crystalloid administration, which worsens certain injuries, such as blast lung, whereas underresuscitation can exacerbate tissue injuries. These pitfalls emphasize the importance of goal-directed fluid resuscitation strategies in the pediatric blast victim.[60]

ETHICS

Making decisions regarding when to potentially withhold or limit treatment in children is emotionally charged and is ethically challenging. However, given the limited resources in disaster settings, health care systems and providers must make these decisions. Incorporating plans for managing ethical dilemmas in pediatric CSC development helps guide hospitals and practitioners in making ethically sound decisions and helps limit provider emotional distress.[61]

The ethical principles that guide practitioners do not change in a disaster. Fairness, duty to care, and duty to steward resources are medical ethical principles that may come into conflict during a disaster when the provider's obligation to the patient competes with their obligation to society. The processes for establishing ethical standards during disasters should have transparency, consistency, proportionality, and accountability.[10]

When crisis standards are used to manage a disaster, scarce resources are allocated to those patients who are most likely to benefit. This egalitarian principle is slightly different from utilitarianism, which seeks to provide care for as many people as possible. There is no universally applicable model that will serve as the definitive resource allocation guide in every situation.[61] Efforts to include a multidisciplinary team in pediatric CSC plans shifts the basis for medical decision-making during disasters from subjective assessments to more objective and evidence-based criteria particularly when dealing with children.[10]

SUMMARY

Children comprise greater than 20% of the US population and tend to be disproportionally injured in disasters but the resources allocated toward children in disaster planning, although improving, are still limited. Children have many inherent developmental, anatomic, and physiologic vulnerabilities, which become more manifest in disaster situations and impact their medical care and systemic needs. It is vital to include children's issues and needs while developing disaster plans including during CSC development, regional patient distribution plans, supply allocation, and treatment pathways.

REFERENCES

1. Dziuban EJ, Peacock G, Frogel M. A child's health is the public's health: progress and gaps in addressing pediatric needs in public health emergencies. Am J Public Health 2017;107(S2):S134–7.

2. Pape JW, Rouzier V, Ford H, et al. The GHESKIO field hospital and clinics after the earthquake in Haiti: dispatch 3 from Port-au-Prince. N Engl J Med 2010. https://doi.org/10.1056/NEJMpv1001787.

3. AAP Disaster Preparedness Advisory Council Committee on Pediatric Emergency Medicine. Ensuring the health of children in disasters. Pediatrics 2015; 136(5):e1407–17.

4. Federal Emergency Management Agency. Children and disasters. Available at: https://www.fema.gov/children-and-disasters. Accessed December 4, 2018.

5. Chamberlain JM, Krug S, Shaw KN. Emergency care for children in the United States. Health Aff (Millwood) 2013;32(12):2109–15.

6. National Commission on Children and Disasters. 2010 Report to the President and Congress. 2010. Available at: https://archive.ahrq.gov/prep/nccdreport/nccdreport.pdf. Accessed March 28, 2018.

7. Save the children. Still at risk: U.S. Children 10 years after hurricane Katrina: 2015 national report card on protecting children in disasters. Available at: https://www.savethechildren.org/content/dam/usa/reports/emergency-prep/disaster-report-2015.pdf. Accessed December 4, 2018.

8. Gausche-Hill M, Ely M, Schmuhl P, et al. A national assessment of pediatric readiness of emergency departments. JAMA Pediatr 2015;169(6):527–34.

9. Lyle KC, Milton J, Fagbuyi D, et al. Pediatric disaster preparedness and response and the nation's children's hospitals. Am J Disaster Med 2015;10(2):83–91.

10. Altevogt BM, Stroud C, Hanson SL, et al. Guidance for establishing crisis standards of care for use in disaster situations: a letter report. Washington, DC: The National Academies Press; 2009.

11. Dries D, Reed MJ, Kissoon N, et al. Special populations. Chest 2014;146(4): e75S–86S.

12. Auf Der Heide E. The importance of evidence-based disaster planning. Ann Emerg Med 2006. https://doi.org/10.1016/j.annemergmed.2005.05.009.

13. Christian MD, Toltzis P, Kanter RK, et al. Treatment and triage recommendations for pediatric emergency mass critical care. Pediatr Crit Care Med 2011;12(6 suppl):109–19.

14. Gall C, Wetzel R, Kolker A, et al. Pediatric triage in a severe pandemic: maximizing survival by establishing triage thresholds. Crit Care Med 2016;44(9): 1762–8.

15. Kanter RK. Strategies to improve pediatric disaster surge response: potential mortality reduction and tradeoffs. Crit Care Med 2007;35(12):2837–42.

16. Hamele M, Poss WB, Sweney J. Disaster preparedness, pediatric considerations in primary blast injury, chemical, and biological terrorism. World J Crit Care Med 2014;3(1):15–23.

17. Barfield WD, Krug SE, Kanter RK, et al. Neonatal and pediatric regionalized systems in pediatric emergency mass critical care. Pediatr Crit Care Med 2011;12(6 SUPPL). https://doi.org/10.1097/PCC.0b013e318234a723.

18. Bohn D, Kanter RK, Burns J, et al. Supplies and equipment for pediatric emergency mass critical care. Pediatr Crit Care Med 2011;12(6 Suppl). https://doi.org/10.1097/PCC.0b013e318234a6b9.

19. Burnett MW, Spinella PC, Azarow KS, et al. Pediatric care as part of the US army medical mission in the global war on terrorism in Afghanistan and Iraq, December 2001 to December 2004. Pediatrics 2008. https://doi.org/10.1007/978-3-0348-0454-7.

20. Tosh PK, Feldman H, Christian MD, et al. Business and continuity of operations: care of the critically ill and injured during pandemics and disasters: CHEST consensus statement. Chest 2014;146:e103S–17S.

21. Custer JW, Watson CM, Dwyer J, et al. Critical evaluation of emergency stockpile ventilators in an. Pediatr Crit Care Med 2011;12(6):357–61.

22. Dominguez-Cherit G, De La Torre A, Rishu A, et al. Influenza a (H1N1pdm09)-related critical illness and mortality in Mexico and Canada, 2014. Crit Care Med 2016;44(10):1861–70.

23. Yung M, Slater A, Festa M, et al. Pandemic H1N1 in children requiring intensive care in Australia and New Zealand during Winter 2009. Pediatrics 2011;127(1): e156–63.

24. Michaels AJ, Hill JG, Bliss D, et al. Pandemic flu and the sudden demand for ECMO resources: a mature trauma program can provide surge capacity in acute critical care crises. J Trauma Acute Care Surg 2013;74(6):1493–7.

25. Vanholder R, Borniche D, Claus S, et al. When the earth trembles in the Americas: the experience of Haiti and Chile 2010. Nephron Clin Pract 2011;117(3). https://doi.org/10.1159/000320200.

26. Wise RA. The creation of emergency health care standards for catastrophic events. Acad Emerg Med 2006;13(11):1150–2.

27. Hota S, Fried E, Burry L, et al. Preparing your intensive care unit for the second wave of H1N1 and future surges. Crit Care Med 2010;38(SUPPL. 4):1–10.

28. Einav S, Hick JL, Hanfling D, et al. Surge capacity logistics: care of the critically ill and injured during pandemics and disasters: chest consensus statement. Chest 2014;146:e17S–43S.

29. American Board of Pediatrics Inc. 2015-2016 workforce data. Chapel Hill (NC): American Board of Pediatrics Inc.; 2016.

30. Grock A, Aluisio AR, Abram E, et al. Evaluation of the association between disaster training and confidence in disaster response among graduate medical trainees: a cross-sectional study. Am J Disaster Med 2017;12(1):5–9.

31. Sprung CL, Zimmerman JL, Christian MD, et al. Recommendations for intensive care unit and hospital preparations for an influenza epidemic or mass disaster: summary report of the European Society of Intensive Care Medicine's Task Force for intensive care unit triage during an influenza epidemic or mas. Intensive Care Med 2010;36(3):428–43.

32. Wallace DJ, Angus DC, Seymour CW, et al. Critical care bed growth in the United States: a comparison of regional and national trends. Am J Respir Crit Care Med 2015;191(4):410–6.

33. Odetola FO, Clark SJ, Freed GL, et al. A national survey of pediatric critical care resources in the United States. Pediatrics 2005;115(4):e382–6.

34. Kanter RK, Moran JR. Pediatric hospital and intensive care unit capacity in regional disasters: expanding capacity by altering standards of care. Pediatrics 2007;119(1):94–100.

35. Flynn-O'Brien KT, Trelles M, Dominguez L, et al. Surgery for children in low-income countries affected by humanitarian emergencies from 2008 to 2014: the Médecins Sans Frontières Operations Centre Brussels experience. J Pediatr Surg 2016;51(4):659–69.

36. Lowe JJ, Gibbs SG, Schwedhelm SS, et al. Nebraska Biocontainment Unit perspective on disposal of Ebola medical waste. Am J Infect Control 2014; 42(12):1256–7.

37. Mason KE, Urbansky H, Crocker L, et al. Pediatric emergency mass critical care: focus on family-centered care. Pediatr Crit Care Med 2011;12(6 SUPPL). https://doi.org/10.1097/PCC.0b013e318234a812.

38. Ratnapalan S, Martimianakis MA, Cohen-Silver JH, et al. Pandemic management in a pediatric hospital. Clin Pediatr (Phila) 2013;52(4):322–8.

39. Barthel ER, Pierce JR, Goodhue CJ, et al. Can a pediatric trauma center improve the response to a mass casualty incident? J Trauma Acute Care Surg 2012;73(4): 885–9.

40. Todd R. Reuniting families after Katrina. CBS News. Available at: http://www.cbsnews.com/stories/2005/09/15/scitech/pcanswer/main850384.shtml. Accessed November 13, 2018.

41. Blake N, Stevenson K. Reunification: keeping families together in crisis. J Trauma 2009;67(SUPPL. 2):147–51.

42. Lowe CG. Pediatric and neonatal interfacility transport medicine after mass casualty incidents. J Trauma 2009;67(SUPPL. 2):168–71.

43. King MA, Niven AS, Beninati W, et al. Evacuation of the ICU. Chest 2014;146(4): e44S–60S.

44. Tegtmeyer K, Conway EE, Upperman JS, et al. Education in a pediatric emergency mass critical care setting. Pediatr Crit Care Med 2011;12(6 SUPPL): 135–40.

45. Mortelmans LJ, Maebe S, Dieltiens G, et al. Are tertiary care paediatricians prepared for disaster situations? Prehosp Disaster Med 2016;31(2):126–31.

46. Society of Critical Care Medicine. Pediatric fundamentals of critical care support. 3rd edition. Mt Prospect (IL): Society for Critical Care Medicine; 2018.

47. Agency for Toxic Substance and Disease Registry. Case studies in environmental medicine: principles of pediatric environmental health. U.S. Department of Health and Human Services; 2006.

48. American Academy of Pediatrics. In: Foltin GL, Schonfeld DJ, Shannon MW, editors. Pediatric disaster preparedness: a resource for pediatricians. Rockville (MD): AHRQ; 2006.

49. Hazinski M. Nursing care for the critically ill child. 3rd edition. Mosby; 2013.

50. Schonfeld DJ, Demaria T. Providing psychosocial support to children and families in the aftermath of disasters and crises. Pediatrics 2015;136(4):e1120–30.

51. Kousky C. Impacts of natural disasters on children. Future Child 2016;26(1): 73–92.

52. Michael WS, Julia AM, Committee on Environmental Health, Committee on Infectious Diseases. Chemical-Biological terrorism and its impact on children. Pediatrics 2006;118(3):1267–78.

53. Vale JA, Marrs TC OBE, Maynard RL CBE. Novichok: a murderous nerve agent attack in the UK. Clin Toxicol 2018;56(11):1093–7.

54. Fuenfer M. Pediatric surgery and medicine for hostile environments; chemical, biological, radiological, nuclear, and explosive injuries. In: Fuenfer M, editor. Washington, DC: Department of Defense, Office of the Surgeon General; 2011. p. 465–89.

55. Weinstein R. Should remaining stockpiles of smallpox virus (Variola) be destroyed? Emerg Infect Dis 2011;17(4):681–3.

56. Tseng CP, Chan Y. Overview of Ebola virus disease in 2014. J Chin Med Assoc 2015;78(1):51–5.

57. American Academy of Pediatrics Committee on Environmental Health. Radiation disasters and children. Pediatrics 2003;11(6):1455–66.

58. Department of the Army, the Navy, the Air Force and CMC. Treatment of nuclear and radiological casualties 2001. Washington, DC.

59. Distribution of attack types used in acts of terrorism worldwide in 2017. Statista. Available at: https://www.statista.com/statistics/622492/attack-types-used-terrorist-attacks-worldwide/. Accessed January 2, 2019.

60. Joseph JW, Sanchez LD. Introduction to explosions and blasts. In: Ciottone GR, editor. Ciottone's disaster medicine. Philadephia: Elsevier; 2015.

61. Hamele M, Neumayer K, Sweney J, et al. Always ready, always prepared: preparing for the next pandemic. Transl Pediatr 2018;7(4):344–55.

Special Populations
Disaster Care Considerations in Chronically Ill, Pregnant, and Morbidly Obese Patients

Timothy M. Dempsey, MD, MPH[a], Stephanie C. Lapinsky, BSc, MD[b],
Eric Melnychuk, DO[c], Stephen E. Lapinsky, MB BCh, MSc, FRCPC[b],
Mary Jane Reed, MD[c],*, Alexander S. Niven, MD[a]

KEYWORDS

- Critical care • Disasters critical illness • Shelter medicine • Oxygen dependent
- Technology dependent • Dialysis • Pregnancy in disaster • Morbid obesity disaster

KEY POINTS

- Special populations are patients with chronic, complex medical conditions who are at increased risk of morbidity and mortality when normal health care services are disrupted during a disaster.
- These patients present unique challenges to providers and health care systems during a disaster, because they represent a substantial population who may require critical care support and resources at a time when staff and resources are limited.
- Local, state, and federal preparation to meet these patients' needs during a disaster is critical to ensure their ongoing care without further disruption to the health care system.
- Previous disaster response efforts can serve as a framework for future preparation to provide care for special populations in a disaster.

INTRODUCTION

The increasing complexity of modern health care has created a substantial population of patients who require regular, ongoing medical treatments, care assistance, and technical support from the health care system. During a disaster, the staff, services, resources, and infrastructure that support these special patient populations are

Disclosure: The authors have nothing to disclose.
[a] Division of Pulmonary and Critical Care Medicine, Mayo Clinic, 200 First Street Southwest, Rochester, MN 55905, USA; [b] Division of Critical Care Medicine, University of Toronto, 600 University Avenue, #18-214, Toronto, Ontario M5G1X5, Canada; [c] Department of Critical Care Medicine, Geisinger Medical Center, 100 North Academy Avenue, Danville, PA 17821-2037, USA
* Corresponding author.
E-mail address: mreed@geisinger.edu
; @tdemps3 (T.M.D.); @mj17820 (M.J.R.); @niven_alex (A.S.N.)

Crit Care Clin 35 (2019) 677–695
https://doi.org/10.1016/j.ccc.2019.06.010
0749-0704/19/© 2019 Elsevier Inc. All rights reserved.

criticalcare.theclinics.com

frequently disrupted, making them vulnerable to significant morbidity and mortality based on past experiences. Despite these past lessons, planning to meet the health care needs of these special populations during future events remains inadequate.

Special populations are commonly defined as "those patients who may be at increased risk for morbidity and mortality outside a fully functional critical care environment, or who present unique challenges to providers when a full complement of supportive services is not available."[1] Common examples include patients who are chronically hospitalized or individuals who reside in an assisted living facility and rely on caregivers for their activities of daily living. Other resource-intensive populations that may present significant challenges during a disaster because of the specialized services and personnel that they require include patients who are morbidly obese, pregnant, or immune compromised. Patients who are dependent on technology, including dialysis, long-term oxygen therapy, and mechanical ventilation, and those with ventricular assist devices, also have significant infrastructure requirements that can be readily disrupted during an environmental event or terrorist attack. In times of need and if local care resources cannot be reestablished, these patients frequently present to hospitals to meet their chronic care needs during periods when critical care personnel are already delivering contingency or crisis care because of the high volume of critically ill patients.

This article describes the impact of disasters on these special patient populations using recent events as examples. These published experiences and existing local, regional, and national disaster plans provide a framework for future disaster preparation and response and identify areas for improvement in need of further research. Given that this population presents unique challenges to the medical system as a whole, this article includes both broad strategies for special population assistance following a disaster and important considerations in the critical care setting.

DEFINING THE PROBLEM

The US Census Bureau estimates that there were nearly 40 million Americans with a disability in 2015, representing 12.6% of the civilian noninstitutionalized population.[2] The impact of a disaster on these individuals is disproportionate and significant compared with the general population. More than 40% of the New Orleans and Louisiana individuals who did not evacuate before Hurricane Katrina were either physically unable to leave or were caring for a person with a disability. Of these individuals, 34% were trapped in their homes, and 17% waited 3 or more days to be rescued.[3]

This lack of mobility, combined with transportation barriers and infrastructure damage during a disaster, can reduce access to routine specialty health care services. Nearly half of the dialysis patients in the New Orleans region missed at least 1 session during Hurricane Katrina and 1 in 6 missed 3 or more sessions, leading to an increased risk of hospitalization.[4] Similarly, during Hurricane Sandy, nearly 40% of dialysis centers in New York City closed after the storm, including 7 that remained shuttered for months.[5] This situation resulted in increased poststorm mortality and hospitalizations in patients requiring dialysis than would have been expected otherwise.[6]

Most recently, Hurricane Maria in Puerto Rico resulted in a significant increase in deaths related to diseases such as Alzheimer, diabetes, and chronic cardiac conditions according to currently available data.[7] Severe damage to the island's power grid forced patients with chronic illness to purchase generators to power their medical equipment. There are also reports of patients with chronic respiratory failure, out of home oxygen supplies, being denied oxygen at local hospitals because of critical shortages.[7] In other disasters, technology-dependent and resource-intensive patients have been refused shelter in facilities overwhelmed and ill-equipped to support their needs.[8]

Lack of community-based resources results in these special patient populations presenting to hospitals for care if and when transportation and evacuation are available. Delayed access to medical services increases the number of individuals requiring acute or critical care. Disasters can affect the delivery of critical care in many ways, depending on the onset, impact, and duration of the incident. During large-scale, mass-casualty events, critical care space, staff, and resources must frequently be adapted using a surge continuum that allocates these limited resources using a framework of contingency or crisis care.[9] Hospitals must be prepared to maximize all patient care areas and even consider nontraditional locations to care for the critically ill depending on need, with current planning recommendations supporting a surge capacity of up to 200%. To meet this goal, bed availability must be enhanced by discharging as many patients as is deemed safe, and available critical care staff and critical care resources increased by at least 100% and strategically deployed to best meet patient care demands.[10] Although these principles are logical in theory, in practice, the options to safely and rapidly discharge patients with significant, complex care needs are limited. This limitation leaves hospitals with the significant challenge of caring for large numbers of both acutely ill patients and medically complex special populations with limited resources.

The documented tragedies from recent natural disaster events in the United States and the challenges of both transporting and caring for medically complex special populations in the community in this setting underline the importance of collaborative planning and preparation by hospitals, local aid agencies, governments, and other organizations or facilities that care for these unique patient groups during a disaster.

SPECIAL POPULATION PLANNING AND CARE

Although detailed considerations of the planning and care of all diverse special populations exceed the scope of this brief review, it identifies important considerations and specific guidance when available for the most common types of patients that intensivists may encounter during disaster response planning or clinical activities after a significant natural event (**Table 1**).

Chronically Hospitalized Patients

Complex care coordination can be a significant barrier to hospital discharge in anticipation of and during disaster events. Special population patients frequently require specific durable medical equipment, nondurable medical supplies, and education or access to skilled health care personnel or facilities to deliver life-sustaining treatments, including dialysis, chronic mechanical ventilation, oxygen therapy, or enteral nutrition. Special medical needs shelters, 8 of which were set up in New York during Superstorm Sandy, offer one solution to this problem.[5] These shelters were developed with the staffing and resources to temporarily care for individuals with significant, chronic needs, including home mechanical ventilation, oxygen, and insulin therapy for diabetics. During the hurricane, they were staffed with hospital personnel consisting of doctors, nurses, and medical assistants. One shelter was open for more than 20 days following the storm and housed up to 175 patients.[5] Enterprising solutions such as special medical needs shelters are essential but do not happen overnight. Without deliberate planning and preparation by city, state, and federal agencies, these services will not be readily available during a disaster.

Table 1
Special patient populations: planning and care

	Planning Phase	Response Phase
Chronically Hospitalized	• Need for complex care coordination	• Space availability in medical needs shelters
Chronic Care Facilities	• Evacuate or not? • Infrastructure concerns	• Dependent on staff for basic care needs • Infrastructure concerns
Technology Dependent	• Insurance coverage for backup supplies (oxygen, batteries) • Patient, caregiver training • Integrated primary care team engagement	• Daily supply, medication requirements • Physical limitations • Need for specialized diets • Need for laboratory monitoring • Specially trained staff • Additional load on stressed system
Oxygen Dependent	• Staff training in basic oxygen equipment • Improve delivery system inefficiencies	• Large-volume compressors, liquid oxygen suppliers preferred • Oxygen-conserving delivery devices
Ventricular Assist Device Dependent	• Early evacuation	• Access to power outlets • Dehydration • Infection risk
Chronic Dialysis Patients	• Preemptive dialysis planning, education	• Coordination services to match dialysis center availability, patient needs
Resource Intensive (Immunosuppressed, Transplant Patients, End-stage Chronic Disease)	• Patient, caregiver training • Integrated primary care team engagement, including pharmacy expertise	• Possible need for isolation infrastructure, increased hygiene, masks • Pharmacy expertise
Pregnant	• Integrated obstetric and neonatal care team engagement	• Possible need for fetal monitoring • Preparation for delivery • Proper positioning, image shielding • Rh prophylaxis
Morbid Obesity	• Staff training in specialized evacuation and transport requirements • Increased supply of decontamination consumables	• Need for specialized equipment for additional weight • Plan for alternative imaging

Chronic Care Facility Residents

Patients in chronic care facilities, as with the chronically hospitalized, are mostly dependent on health care staff for assistance. Although the Centers for Medicare and Medicaid Services (CMS) mandates that nursing homes and long-term care facilities have an emergency preparedness plan, prior disasters have shown such policies to be inadequate. During both Hurricanes Katrina and Sandy, local authorities decided not to evacuate nursing homes. Ultimately, 215 nursing home residents died during Katrina, and infrastructure damage (including failed generators) forced the National Guard to rescue more than 4000 nursing home residents during Sandy.[5,11] Many of these patients ended up in special medical needs shelters, hospitals, and intensive care units (ICUs), requiring the assistance of essential staff and using vital resources that could have been used elsewhere had appropriate local facility planning occurred.

The decision to shelter in place during a disaster is reasonable, given studies showing increased mortality for nursing home patients following evacuation.[12] However, past events underline the importance of anticipatory planning and response to fundamental infrastructure failures to reduce the risk of harm to an already vulnerable nursing home population during a disaster. Local regulators declared 12 of the 14 deaths that occurred in a Florida nursing home following a power outage during Hurricane Irma homicides, leading regulators to revoke the responsible facility's license.[12] More than a year after the hurricane, up to three-quarters of Florida nursing homes are still without generators that meet state requirements.[13] Although current consensus statements recommend all health care facilities develop a detailed evacuation plan and simulation exercises for chronically ill patients, only 1 in 3 nursing home emergency preparedness plans include an evacuation route.[14–16]

Lessons from prior disasters have proved useful to better care for chronic care patients moving forward. Hurricane Katrina prompted improved communication and partnership between state agencies and nursing homes, and nursing home directors reported they were significantly more confident in their preparations to manage Hurricane Gustav, which hit Louisiana 3 years after Katrina.[17] A detailed disaster plan developed collaboratively between nursing homes and emergency services has also been shown to improve outcomes in a public health emergency.[18] As with chronically hospitalized patients, the importance of integrating nursing home planning into local, state, and federal disaster preparation is imperative.

Technology-dependent Patients

Patients dependent on technology, including home oxygen, chronic mechanical ventilation, ventricular assist devices (VADs), enteral feeding, and dialysis, can create a strain on both hospitals and shelters during disasters. There are several common barriers and solutions that the literature regularly identifies in the planning and response phases for the care of these patients. Insurance coverage for additional durable medical equipment items (ie, oxygen tanks, VAD batteries) can be challenging to obtain, making prepositioning of backup resources difficult. Training patients and caregivers to provide self-care, engaging primary care teams in disaster planning efforts to provide additional assistance, and identifying special medical needs shelters are potential solutions that could be better leveraged.[1]

Although these specialized shelters offered a promising solution during Hurricane Sandy, they involve challenges. Common issues include restocking of medical supplies and medications, managing patients with significant physical limitations, meeting specialized diet requirements, and providing necessary laboratory monitoring. These issues can present significant barriers to care and underline the importance of deliberate staff training, medication adherence programs, and physical space planning for essential elements such as appropriate electrical outlets to ensure successful patient outcomes.[1] Some experts recommend that patients with similar medical requirements (ie, oxygen therapy) should be clustered to make it easier for staff to provide appropriate care.

There are several important issues associated with specific technology-dependent populations that are important to review.

Oxygen-dependent patients

Oxygen is perhaps the most crucial consumable medical resource during a disaster.[19] Without it, many patients with chronic lung diseases experience significant setbacks, resulting in increases in emergency room visits, hospital admissions, and further strain on an already burdened system. During the 2011 earthquake in Japan, one hospital reported a 20% exacerbation rate among the 83 patients with chronic lung disease requiring oxygen soon after the event.[20] The addition of a large number of oxygen-dependent patients to a strained hospital system can present a significant problem when supply chains are disrupted. Ritz and Previtera[21] found that their 385-bed hospital (with 65 ICU beds) uses 1703 L (450 gallons) of liquid oxygen (1.5 million gaseous liters) per day. Although the Strategic National Stockpile, a federal agency maintained by the Department of Health and Human Services, delivers pharmaceuticals and medical supplies for use in an emergency, it relies on private vendor contracts to distribute backup oxygen tanks, which may prove an unreliable resource in a disaster.[19] For individuals, one possibility is the use of oxygen-conserving devices such as reservoir nasal cannula to help reduce demands.[1] For hospitals and shelters, larger-capacity concentrators and liquid oxygen delivery systems are good options for supporting bulk delivery.[19] Other recommendations include easy access to bulk oxygen delivery areas, staff education in basic oxygen tank handling and refilling, regular wall outlet checks for leaks, and shutting off unused meters that do not routinely require oxygen supplementation.

Patients with ventricular assist devices

VADs are crucial life support equipment that may stress an already strained health care infrastructure during a public health emergency. Battery life must be supported at all times. A strict diet and medication regimen must be adhered to as well. Disaster concerns for these patients include power outages, limited access to medications, dehydration, and conditions that may increase the risk for infection.[22] Although medication adherence programs, diet modifications, and ensuring electrical outlet access should be performed whenever possible, these patients may ultimately end up overwhelming an already beleaguered system. There are reports of the systematic evacuation of VAD patients during a disaster, which may be considered if necessary.[23]

Patients with end-stage renal disease on dialysis

During disasters, the closure of dialysis centers in affected regions (sometimes for as long as months) has resulted in increased hospitalizations for patients with end-stage renal disease (ESRD).[6] Earthquakes may both increase the need for acute dialysis because of crush injuries and compromise hospital and intensive care unit clean water supplies, further compromising the ability to meet renal replacement therapy requirements.[24,25] In some settings, urgent dialysis volumes have forced patients with less severe hyperkalemia to be temporized with medications rather than renal replacement.[24] Other sites have relied on shorter dialysis runs to maximize the number of people who can receive benefit from this intervention.[5]

The ESRD Network of New York, a group commissioned by CMS to guarantee the availability of emergency preparedness services to dialysis patients in the state, successfully used a multipronged strategy before, during, and after Hurricane Sandy to (1) provide patients with contact information and newsletters about where to go before the event; (2) instruct patients on a modified diet during the emergency; (3) set up emergency phone services during and after the hurricane; (4) ensure that dialysis centers provided extended hours before the hurricane; and (5) make sure patients received sessions just before the storm, even if they were not due.[5] Such a forward-thinking approach in both the planning and response phases offers an excellent model for future events.

Resource-intensive Populations

Other resource-intensive populations that require special attention during disasters include the immune compromised, transplant patients, and others with end-stage chronic diseases such as cirrhosis. These individuals also require careful predisaster planning, education, and coordination with caregivers and primary care providers, as well as identification of special medical needs shelters that can meet their care requirements in situ. During the disaster, they also require a medication adherence program, diet modification, and specially trained staff. Unique to this population is the possible need for isolation (regardless of space constraints) to protect them from the potential harmful conditions within shelters or hospitals during a public health emergency. Masks and hand hygiene are also critically important. During Hurricane Sandy an infection prevention specialist was deployed at a specific medical needs shelter to help ensure adherence to appropriate hygiene practices and effectively prevented outbreaks of bed bugs, upper respiratory infections, and gastrointestinal issues at one shelter during the crisis.[26]

Pregnancy

Women and children may be disproportionately affected by natural disasters, and women likely have a higher mortality than men.[27] A study of patients managed in a field hospital in the first 14 days after the 2010 earthquake in Haiti identified that 10% of patients were pregnant and 20% of these delivered.[28] Of pregnant women hospitalized for trauma, 5% to 24% deliver during that hospitalization, most within 24 hours of injury.[29] Immunologic changes in pregnancy may affect susceptibility to certain infectious conditions; for example, influenza. In the influenza epidemic of 1957, half of the fatalities among women of childbearing age occurred in pregnant women.[30] Pregnant women represent a unique population in the ICU and in disaster situations for reasons that are discussed here briefly.

Altered physiology and immunology in pregnancy Pregnant women undergo physiologic changes affecting various systems relevant to their assessment and management in a disaster situation, in particular the respiratory, cardiovascular, and immune systems. Respiratory changes include edema and hyperemia of the upper airways caused by hormonal effects, making endotracheal intubation more difficult.[31] Intubation usually requires a smaller tube and should be managed by the most expert operator available. Although total lung capacity changes only minimally, a 10% to 25% decrease in functional residual capacity occurs.[32] This reduction in the oxygen reservoir, combined with an increased oxygen consumption (by 33% above baseline), causes pregnant women to desaturate rapidly in the presence of lung disease or apnea.[33] Tidal volume and minute ventilation increase, resulting in a mild respiratory alkalosis with compensatory renal excretion of bicarbonate ($Paco_2$ 28–32 mm Hg; HCO_3^- 18–21 mEq/L).

Cardiac output is increased during pregnancy, reaching 30% to 50% above baseline by 28 weeks.[34] Blood flow to the uterus increases dramatically during pregnancy, from about 50 mL/min to almost 1000 mL/min by term,[35] putting pregnant patients at risk of sudden and catastrophic blood loss. In the supine position, the enlarged uterus may obstruct venous return from the inferior vena cava (and from the placenta), potentially causing maternal hypotension and fetal distress(the supine hypotensive syndrome).[36]

Pregnant women's immune systems are altered to allow tolerance to paternally derived fetal antigens. This process occurs by downregulation of cell-mediated immunity, balanced by upregulation of the humoral immune response.[37,38] The net effect is a predisposition to more severe manifestations of certain infections usually prevented by cell-mediated immunity, including viral and fungal infections. Pregnant women also seem to be more susceptible to developing acute respiratory distress syndrome (ARDS) than nonpregnant patients, related to an immunologic effect as well as the increased circulating blood volume and hypoalbuminemia. The lungs may be primed for the development of ARDS by inflammatory changes resulting from the process of labor and delivery.[39]

Altered manifestations of trauma in pregnant women Pregnant patients with trauma should be treated similarly to their nonpregnant counterparts, but with attention to some significant differences in presentation and management. Premature labor can occur in up to 25% of trauma cases with gestation beyond 22 weeks.[40] Severe maternal hemorrhage may occur as a result of uterine trauma, because of the high uterine blood flow. Blunt trauma can, in rare cases, result in uterine rupture, and penetrating injury to the abdomen in later pregnancy most commonly affects the uterus.[41] Penetrating injury may also result in significant damage to intra-abdominal viscera, which are compressed in the upper abdomen. Fracture of the pelvis can result in severe retroperitoneal hemorrhage because of the dilated pelvic veins.

Fetal loss may occur as a result of maternal shock or hypoxia, placental injury, or because of direct injury to the fetus. Placental abruption is an important cause of fetal demise following maternal trauma, and may be complicated by disseminated intravascular coagulopathy caused by release of thromboplastin into the maternal circulation. Abruption may present with vaginal bleeding, uterine tenderness or abdominal cramps, amniotic fluid leakage, and unexplained fetal distress or maternal hypovolemia. Blunt trauma may produce fetal head injury often related to maternal pelvic fracture. Maternal burns to greater than 30% of the body surface area result in a high fetal mortality.

Evaluation of pregnant patients with trauma should note that physical signs may be altered by changing organ position and by the reduced peritoneal sensitivity in pregnancy. Obstetric consultation and fetal monitoring are important when the fetus is at a viable gestation. Continuous fetal heart rate monitoring is the optimal method for identifying uteroplacental insufficiency or abruption after trauma. Approximately 80% of abruption occurs in the first 6 hours, with the remaining 20% occurring within 24 hours after injury.[29] Continuous electronic fetal monitoring is therefore usually recommended for the first 4 to 6 hours. Ultrasonography is used for evaluation of the fetus for injury and biophysical profile, and to assess for intra-abdominal organ damage. Transplacental hemorrhage of fetal blood into the maternal circulation may occur in about 10% to 30% of pregnant patients with trauma.[42] This hemorrhage can cause fetal exsanguination into the maternal circulation and also maternal Rh sensitization. Fetal red cells may be identified in the maternal blood smear (Kleihauer-Betke test), confirming the presence of fetomaternal hemorrhage and also permitting an estimate of the volume of red cells of fetal origin. Maternal blood type and Rh status should be assessed, noting that specimens for crossmatch must be renewed every 72 hours because of the possibility of development of alloantibodies during pregnancy.

Management efforts directed at stabilizing the mother are beneficial to both mother and fetus. Fluid replacement may need to be given more rapidly in pregnant women because of the increase in plasma volume in pregnancy. Maternal heart rate and blood pressure may not be reliable predictors of the degree of hemorrhage. Prevention of the supine hypotensive syndrome requires positioning on the left side. All Rh-negative mothers with abdominal trauma should receive Rh immune globulin, and, if significant fetomaternal hemorrhage occurs (quantified by the Kleihauer-Betke test), higher doses of Rh immune globulin are required.

Fetal risk and maternal critical illness During critical illness, the fetus is at risk from therapeutic and diagnostic interventions performed on the mother, as well as from the effects of maternal disease.

A major concern that commonly arises is the risk to the fetus from radiological investigations. The risk to the fetus is very low and necessary maternal investigations should not be withheld. The effects of radiation on the fetus include teratogenicity, effects on neurologic development, and an increased risk of childhood leukemia, depending on the gestation of exposure. However, these effects require radiation doses in the range of 50 to 200 mGy, far higher than the fetal exposure from most diagnostic radiographic investigations.[43] For example, a well-shielded maternal chest radiograph exposes the fetus to about 0.01 mGy and a chest computed tomography (CT) scan to about 0.66 mGy.[44] In contrast, a CT scan of the mother's abdomen and pelvis (as may be required following maternal trauma) exposes the fetus to up to 50 mGy with a potential increased risk of childhood leukemia.[45] In contrast with medical X-ray exposure, maternal accidental radiation exposure (eg, atomic bombs) is associated with significant neurologic developmental problems and cancer risk in offspring.[43]

Pharmacologic therapy during pregnancy should consider the altered pharmacokinetics (altered volume of distribution, renal clearance), the effect of some drugs on uterine and placental perfusion, and teratogenic effects. The uteroplacental vascular bed is usually maximally dilated, and alpha-adrenergic agonists may markedly decrease blood flow.[46] Although most vasoactive infusions (eg, norepinephrine, epinephrine) tend to reduce uterine blood flow and potentially impair fetal oxygen delivery, these drugs should be used when lifesaving for the mother. Teratogenicity should not influence drug therapy in critically ill mothers, but unnecessary pharmacotherapy should be avoided. The Food and Drug Administration (FDA) of the United States has warned that prolonged or repeated administration of general anesthetic or sedative drugs to pregnant women during the third trimester may affect the development of the fetal brain.[47] This statement was based largely on animal studies; human data are sparse and inconclusive, and this statement generated considerable controversy.

Partial pressure of oxygen in the umbilical vein (returning from the placenta to the fetus) is about 28 mm Hg.[45] Fetal oxygenation is therefore precarious, and depends on maternal oxygenation and placental perfusion. A decrease in maternal oxygen saturation is likely to cause a significant decrease in fetal oxygen delivery.[48] No good human data are available to identify the adverse effects of acute maternal hypoxia on fetuses. Clinical practice is usually to aim for a maternal oxygen saturation greater than 92% to 95%(Pao_2 70 mm Hg) when possible, although evidence to support this threshold is lacking.

Unique indications for intensive care unit admission ICU admission in pregnant women is required for a variety of causes, with no significant differences between low-resource and high-resource countries.[49] ICU admission is required in about 0.3% of pregnancies. The most common reasons for ICU admission are the hypertensive disorders of pregnancy (30%–40% of admissions of pregnant women), followed by obstetric hemorrhage (20%–25%).[49] Other causes include sepsis (5%), other obstetric complications (5%), and various other causes unrelated to the pregnancy (eg, pneumonia, trauma).

A review of obstetric conditions resulting in ICU admission is beyond the scope of this article, but it is important in disaster planning to consider the expertise, equipment, and drugs that may be required. Preeclampsia is a pregnancy-specific hypertensive disorder affecting approximately 3% to 10% of pregnancies, and is associated with several complications necessitating ICU management.[50] These complications include hypertensive crises such as pulmonary edema with respiratory failure, intracerebral hemorrhage, and renal failure. Eclampsia is the occurrence of seizures in a preeclamptic woman, not attributable to other causes. Thrombocytopenia and microangiopathic hemolytic anemia may complicate preeclampsia, and the HELLP (hemolysis, elevated liver enzymes, and low platelet count) syndrome implies this combination in addition to acute hepatic dysfunction.[51] A marked coagulopathy in a peripartum women requires significant resources to manage successfully. Management of preeclampsia requires antihypertensive therapy, and older drugs are most commonly used in pregnancy because of their safety profiles. Oral drugs commonly used include methyldopa, hydralazine, labetalol, and nifedipine, whereas labetalol and hydralazine are used intravenously. Magnesium sulfate is a lifesaving drug in this situation and should always be available. It is used intramuscularly (eg, 6–10 g loading and 2–4 g every 4 hours) or intravenously (eg, 4 g loading and 1–2 g/h infusion) for prophylaxis and for treatment of eclamptic seizures.[52] Magnesium toxicity (common in the presence of renal failure) may cause heart block and respiratory muscle weakness.

Obstetric hemorrhage is a common and potentially life-threatening complication of delivery. Management requires obstetric expertise and access to blood and blood products. The early use of tranexamic acid improves outcomes and has become standard practice.[53] Certain drugs and equipment may be requested by obstetricians; for example, oxytocin, ergometrine, carboprost, and misoprostol, as well as packing, retractors, sutures, and intrauterine tamponade balloons. Interventional radiology and surgical intervention may become necessary.

Obstetric delivery Appropriate expertise and necessary drugs and equipment for delivery should be easily accessible in the ICU for any critically ill pregnant woman with a fetus at a viable gestation. Premature delivery may be precipitated by trauma or other critical illness, or may be necessitated by sudden fetal compromise. Equipment for vaginal delivery, cesarean delivery, and for neonatal resuscitation should be available near the bedside, as well as contact details for obstetric and neonatal support. Fetal viability and resuscitation status should be established ahead of time, the gestation of viability being determined by patient's values as well as the availability of neonatal intensive care services, which may be compromised in a disaster situation.

In mechanically ventilated patients, some improvement in oxygenation or compliance may occur with delivery, but not necessarily in all patients.[54] Women with an obstetric cause for respiratory failure are more likely to benefit from delivery than those with nonobstetric causes.[55] The decision to deliver requires multidisciplinary input, including critical care, maternal-fetal medicine, and neonatology, and the mode of delivery is based on usual obstetric principles.

In a resource-limited situation, gestational age is likely to be based on dating by last menstrual period. Management of delivery in a disaster comes with several unique challenges. Experience from the 2010 Haitian earthquake report describes 12 deliveries in 60 pregnant women, all by vaginal delivery using active management of labor with oxytocin infusion and analgesia with subcutaneous morphine.[2] Cesarean section, with the associated immobility and risk of complications, including bleeding and infection, was avoided. Zidovudine was available if human immunodeficiency virus infection was identified and all infants received vitamin K intramuscularly and erythromycin eye ointment. $Rh_o(D)$ immune globulin was not available. Other disaster reports describe a high incidence of premature delivery and neonatal morbidity, and sanitary challenges with neonatal tetanus from cord cutting in a contaminated environment.[2] To facilitate the risk stratification and to develop a universal language for obstetric-specific triage, the OB TRAIN (Obstetric Triage by Resource Allocation for Inpatient) system has been developed, with an antepartum and a postpartum algorithm.[56] This system identifies the type of transport and accompaniment required for obstetric patients undergoing regional evacuation. A valuable, free, on-line resource for general information on management of pregnant women is the Global Library of Women's Medicine.[57]

Morbidly obese patients

Severe (morbid) obesity is defined as a body mass index of 40 kg/m^2 or higher, and its prevalence has been steadily increasing in the Unites States. Morbidly obese people affected by disasters present unique challenges in several aspects of their care. Several cases have been published about the challenges in caring for these patients in disaster settings.[58] Morbidly obese patients are considered a special population according to the US Department of Health and Human Services' National Response Framework and All Hazards Preparedness Act. This special population requires additional needs in maintaining independence, with increased requirements relating to transportation, supervision, and medical care compared with the general population during a disaster.[1]

Comorbidities related to obesity are common and can affect any body system. The most common comorbidities include depression, obstructive sleep apnea, hypertension, dyslipidemia, cardiovascular disease, type 2 diabetes mellitus, chronic kidney disease, and cancer. Presence of these comorbidities may lead to increased reliance and support in the form of medications and medical devices, and may increase the likelihood of these patients experiencing harm in a disaster.[59]

Surgical correction of obesity A patient's history of surgical correction of obesity is an important factor to consider in caring for patients in disasters. The surgical correction of obesity has associated complications, such as marginal ulcers, bowel obstructions, adhesions, and internal and abdominal wall hernias. The signs and symptoms related to these complications may mimic those of disaster-related complications such as blast abdomen; blunt abdominal trauma; and toxin, biological, chemical, or acute radiation exposure. The most common surgical procedures to correct obesity include Roux-en-Y gastric bypass, duodenal switch, gastric sleeve, and gastric banding. Altering the gastrointestinal tract in these surgeries leads to altered nutritional requirements, micronutrient and macronutrient deficiency, and food intolerances.[59]

Transportation Morbid obesity can be a disabling medical condition. As a patient's weight increases, difficulties with mobility escalate. Resources, equipment, and staff required to assist the patient in moving increase. Transportation out of the home or care facility requires specialized apparatus, including large litters, sleds, or chairs, and these must be available and functional for use. Transport vehicle loading may require ramps or winches and other contrivances as well as additional staff to safely transport the patient from home or care facility to ambulance, and ambulance to hospital. In the resource-constrained environments of disasters, normal support and care for this population may be threatened.[58,59]

Transport vehicles typically have weight limitations and may need more fuel and fewer staff able to support the patient because of space restrictions within the vehicle, especially in air transport vehicles. Because of space restrictions in these vehicles, more staff and transport vehicles may be needed to transport nonobese patients in disasters. Obese individuals take up more space in transport vehicles, which may decrease the number of people who can be evacuated at one time in the same transport vehicle.[58,59]

Positional requirements of obese patients in disasters is of importance. Morbidly obese patients have decreased functional residual capacity, expiratory reserve volume, and total lung capacity at baseline. The supine position may lead to further decreased functional residual capacity because of hampered diaphragmatic movement from increased abdominal pressure and decreased chest wall compliance, and is generally uncomfortable for obese patients. Therefore, the reverse Trendelenburg position may be more comfortable for these patients.

Pressure-induced rhabdomyolysis of dependent areas of buttocks and extremities caused by immobility and long transport times is a potential complication. Acute compartment syndrome may develop, and the classic signs of compartment syndrome may not be readily discernible because of increased adipose tissue in these areas. This complication may be more difficult to diagnose if the patient is intubated and sedated and unable to express pain effectively.[59]

Care area equipment and medications Noninvasive blood pressure monitoring, venous access, and airway issues are common in obese patients. A small blood pressure cuff may overestimate blood pressure by up to 50 mm Hg. Therefore, blood pressure cuff bladder length should be 75% to 80% of the upper arm circumference and width should be greater than 50% of the length of the upper arm. Obtaining and interpreting imaging studies in morbidly obese patients can be challenging. Underpenetration of plain radiograph films is common and abdominal ultrasonography as well as echocardiography can be technically difficult and windows may be limited. Weight limitations and limitations in aperture diameter and table thickness in CT and MRI scanners should also be considered. Peripheral vascular access is challenging, even with the assistance of ultrasonography.[1]

The distribution, protein binding, and clearance of medications in morbidly obese patients are different than that of nonobese patients. There is an increased volume of distribution of lipophilic medications and an increased clearance of hydrophilic medications caused by higher metabolic demands than in nonobese patients. Larger quantities of weight-based medications, such as anti-infectives, analgesics, and anti-epileptics, are needed in obese patients and could deplete the emergency medication cache more rapidly. Medications with narrow therapeutic windows, such as anticoagulants, should be used carefully. Medications used for sedation and analgesia in nonintubated patients should also be used carefully because morbidly obese patients may have undiagnosed sleep disturbances, such as sleep apnea, and increased hypercapnia and hypoxemia.[1,59]

The US Department of Health and Human Services maintains several Federal Medical Stations that can deploy at disaster locations. Each Federal Medical Station can deploy an approximate 250-bed capability, which includes 3 days of medical supplies, including medications that are deployed in large, structurally sound buildings in the location of the disaster. The US Department of Health and Human Services has developed a set of supplies that include beds, lifts, walkers, wheelchairs, toilets, continuous positive airway pressure (CPAP) machines, and CPAP masks specifically for obese patients.[59]

Care area space and staff The task force on mass critical care recommends critically ill patients be cared for in hospital settings during disasters as opposed to field hospitals or other settings because of their special needs. During disasters, areas of the hospital may be repurposed to care for the critically ill to increase surge capacity, requiring specialized equipment be available in those areas to care for this population. Staff education on the care of obese patients is important considering the increased support needed to adequately care for these patients along with maintaining empathy, respect, and dignity to the patients. Safety of staff is essential to caring for this population and a team-assist approach should be used to transfer patients who cannot support their own weight.[58,59]

Management of obese patients in specific disasters

Trauma Clinical examination of obese patients with trauma can be unreliable because of skin folds masking penetrating injuries, difficulty auscultating lung and heart sounds, difficulty assessing abdominal and extremity tenderness, masses or deformities, and difficulty with log rolling. The focused assessment with sonography in trauma (FAST) scan may be technically difficult in obese patients with trauma because of beam penetration and image quality and is considered less sensitive in obese patients. Adipose tissue may resemble clotted blood, leading to false-positive subxyphoid views of a pericardial fat pad resembling hemopericardium.[59]

Intubation of obese patients may be complicated by increased parapharyngeal adipose tissue leading to upper airway collapse, decreased lung and chest wall compliance leading to more rapid desaturation while apneic, and increased risk of aspiration caused by increased intra-abdominal pressures and increased gastric volumes. It is important to prepare for intubation adequately, especially with regard to preoxygenation. After intubation, PEEP requirements are typically higher than those of nonobese patients because of decreased chest wall compliance and higher risk of significant atelectasis.[58,59]

Difficulties with central venous and peripheral arterial access under ultrasonography guidance may be present and may require longer catheters to adequately cannulate the intended vessel. Excess adipose tissue at the sites of venous and arterial access should be monitored closely because excess tissue may shift after repositioning and become dislodged. Arterial blood pressure monitoring may be needed because noninvasive means of blood pressure monitoring may be inaccurate, as discussed earlier.[59]

Although evidence is conflicting, obesity in patients with trauma has been associated with higher mortality, longer duration of intubation and mechanical ventilation, increased ICU and hospital length of stay, increased rates of organ dysfunction, and increased complication rates. These findings should be considered in planning support for the obese patients in disasters.[58,59]

Natural disasters Natural disasters are associated with specific injures, such as crush injuries from collapse of structures, lacerations and blunt trauma from falling debris, hypothermia or hyperthermia, and drownings. Obese patients tend to experience longer extraction times because of difficulties with immobility and additional equipment and staff needed for extraction, predisposing them to a higher risk of significant crush injury. Because of the chronic inflammatory state of obesity and poor skin blood flow, wound healing is jeopardized and secondary infections may develop. Time to rewarm and evaporative cooling may be prolonged because of the increased amount of tissue needed to be warmed or cooled in hypothermia and hypothermia, respectively. Obese individuals are more prone to hyperthermia because of poor skin blood flow and increased adipose tissue.[58,59]

Biological, chemical, and radiation exposures The general principles of biological, chemical, and radiation exposures are removal from the contaminated environment, decontamination, provision of reversal agents if appropriate, and supportive care. Because of obese patients' mobility constraints, inability to move out of the contaminated area without assistance may lead to prolonged exposure. Removal of the patient and subsequent decontamination may require specialized equipment and increased staff as previously discussed. Increased dosages of medications may be needed for symptomatic control of certain toxins. Isolation precautions may also be needed in certain biological exposures. Because of the increased staff and equipment needed to transfer or turn patients for basic care, it is likely that disposable personal protective equipment will be depleted at a faster rate.[58,59]

Psychological and psychiatric support In general, the morbidly obese are at higher risk of depression, social isolation, and decreased self-esteem caused by social prejudice. Morbidly obese patients with underlying psychiatric disease require mental health support in the acute phase of disaster as well as during the recovery and rehabilitation phases of injury and/or illness after the disaster. Also important is adequate attention to palliative support, pain management, and preferred nonpharmacologic anxiolysis during disaster.[1,59]

Disaster triage and allocation of resources Under normal circumstances, morbidly obese critically ill patients require more and specialized resources. Morbidly obese patients generally have more comorbidities than nonobese patients; however, patient body mass index or weight status is not part of any current model to triage patients in disasters. A focus on transparency is needed to adequately triage patients in disasters given what resources are available.

A FRAMEWORK FOR PLANNING AND RESPONSE TO DISASTER

Similar strategies have been used to care for special populations in recent disasters, regardless of the medical setting The most successful strategies described in the literature seem to take the following approach (also described in **Box 1**):[1,11,60]

Planning stages
1. Disaster preparedness is incorporated into primary health care management and facility maintenance. This approach was seen during Hurricane Sandy when the ESRD Network of New York developed a multipronged approach to dialysis management in the days leading up to the storm.[5]

Box 1
Framework for disaster planning, response in special populations

Planning phase
1. Disaster preparedness incorporated into primary health care management, facility maintenance
2. Preemptive identification and contingency planning for patients at risk for decompensation before event
3. Integration of community-based organizations in planning process
4. Designation of regionalized specialty centers to handle most complex patients

Response phase
5. Appropriate triage and resource allocation, similar to general population
6. Appropriate transfer to regionalized specialty centers for complex care
7. Clustering of special populations into special medical needs shelters, alternative care facilities
8. Communication between local, state, and federal agencies

2. Proactive identification and contingency planning for patients at risk of decompensation or who require significant assistance can be performed by a multidisciplinary team of local and state agencies, including education and simulation events to improve preparedness.[61] The creation of a central database for patients with advanced needs by either state-based or community-based organizations would also be extremely beneficial.
3. Community-based organizations should be involved in all phases of emergency preparedness planning.
4. Regionalized specialty centers should be identified. These centers receive the most complex patients with the highest level of need during disasters. By concentrating resources, expertise, and planning in specific locations, this strategy has resulted in fewer costs in the past and may also decrease morbidity and mortality.[62]

Response stages

5. Special populations should be appropriately triaged and have resources allocated following the same guidelines and ethical principles as the general population.[63,64]
6. Patients whose needs exceed the capacity of a given ICU, hospital, or shelter should undergo early and appropriate transfer to identified regionalized specialty centers.
7. Special populations who do not require transfer should be clustered into special medical needs shelters or alternative care facilities that will help with hospital overflow and ensure the needs of these patients are met (as previously discussed).
8. Local, state, and federal agencies in charge of response and relief efforts should have continuous communication with nursing homes, shelters, and hospitals during the event.

FUTURE DIRECTIONS

Despite many examples of successful special population care during recent disasters, there remain several areas for further improvement. Additional research is needed on (1) the creation of better systems to identify and support at-risk patients during both planning and response; (2) the best allocation of resources and personnel between hospitals, special medical needs shelters, and other facilities; (3) careful review of the evidence suggesting increased risk associated with the evacuation of chronic care facility residents, shelters, and hospitals in the setting of improved emergency preparedness plans; and (4) the best mechanisms to foster improved collaboration between hospitals and local, state, and federal agencies before, during, and after a disaster.

SUMMARY

Special populations are groups of patients that present unique challenges within the medical system during a disaster and are often overlooked in planning. They require significant attention before, during, and after a public health emergency. This growing population of chronically ill and morbidly obese patients represents an enormous potential threat to overtaxed hospital and ICU resources during surge situations, but is also at risk for significant morbidity and mortality if cared for in places with insufficient resources and infrastructure support. Only through careful preparation and ongoing evaluation of successful practices will the care of this vulnerable group be optimized.

REFERENCES

1. Dries D, Reed MJ, Kissoon N, et al. Special populations: care of the critically ill and injured during pandemics and disasters: CHEST consensus statement. Chest 2014;146(4 Suppl):e75S–86S.

2. United States Census Bureau. 2015 American community survey: disability characteristics 2015. Available at: https://factfinder.census.gov/faces/tableservices/jsf/pages/productview.xhtml?pid=ACS_15_1YR_S1810&prodType=table. Accessed February 5, 2019.

3. Brodie M, Weltzien E, Altman D, et al. Experiences of hurricane Katrina evacuees in Houston shelters: implications for future planning. Am J Public Health 2006;96: 1402–8.

4. Anderson AH, Cohen AJ, Kutner NG, et al. Missed dialysis sessions and hospitalization in hemodialysis patients after Hurricane Katrina. Kidney Int 2009; 75(11):1202–8.

5. Teperman S. Hurricane Sandy and the greater New York health care system. J Trauma Acute Care Surg 2013;74(6):1401–10.

6. Kelman J, Finne K, Bogdanov A, et al. Dialysis care and death following Hurricane Sandy. Am J Kidney Dis 2015;65(1):109–15.

7. Santos-Burgoa C, Sandberg J, Suárez E, et al. Differential and persistent risk of excess mortality from Hurricane Maria in Puerto Rico: a time-series analysis. Lancet Planet Health 2018;2(11):478–88.

8. Nick GA, Saviola E, Elqura L, et al. Emergency preparedness for vulnerable populations: people with special health-care needs. Public Health Rep 2009;124(2): 338–43, 9.

9. Christian MD, Devereaux AV, Dichter JR, et al. Introduction and executive summary: care of the critically ill and injured during pandemics and disasters: CHEST consensus statement. Chest 2014;146(4 Suppl):8s–34s.

10. Lam C, Waldhorn R, Toner E, et al. The prospect of using alternative medical care facilities in an influenza pandemic. Biosecur Bioterror 2006;4(4):384–90.

11. Wingate MS, Perry EC, Campbell PH, et al. Identifying and protecting vulnerable populations in public health emergencies: addressing gaps in education and training. Public Health Rep 2007;122(3):422–6.

12. Alanez T, Pesantes E. 12 nursing home deaths in Hollywood ruled as homicides. South Florida Sun Sentinel 2017.

13. Payne M. Most Florida nursing homes don't have generators despite new requirement after Irma deaths. Fort Myers News-Press. 2018.

14. King MA, Niven AS, Beninati W, et al, on behalf of the Task Force for Mass Critical Care. Evacuation of the ICU. Care of the critically ill and injured during pandemics and disasters: CHEST consensus statement. Chest 2014;146(4 Suppl):e44S–60S.

15. Willoughby M, Kipsaina C, Ferrah N, et al. Mortality in nursing homes following emergency evacuation: a systematic review. J Am Med Dir Assoc 2017;18(8): 664–70.

16. Castle NG. Nursing home evacuation plans. Am J Public Health 2008;98(7): 1235–40.

17. Blanchard G, Dosa D. A comparison of the nursing home evacuation experience between hurricanes Katrina (2005) and Gustav (2008). J Am Med Dir Assoc 2009;10(9):639–43.

18. Koning SW, Ellerbroek PM, Leenen LP. Indoor fire in a nursing home: evaluation of the medical response to a mass casualty incident based on a standardized protocol. Eur J Trauma Emerg Surg 2015;41(2):167–78.

19. Blakeman TC, Branson RD. Oxygen supplies in disaster management. Respir Care 2013;58(1):173–83.
20. Kobayashi S, Hanagama M, Yamanda S, et al. Home oxygen therapy during natural disasters: lessons from the great East Japan earthquake. Eur Respir J 2012; 39(4):1047–8.
21. Ritz RH, Previtera JE. Oxygen supplies during a mass casualty situation. Respir Care 2008;53(2):215–24.
22. Davis KJ, O'Shea G, Beach M. Assessment of risks posed to VAD patients during disasters. Prehosp Disaster Med 2017;32(4):457–61.
23. Owens WR, Morales DL, Braham DG, et al. Hurricane Katrina: emergent interstate transport of an evacuee on biventricular assist device support. ASAIO J 2006;52(5):598–600.
24. Amundson D, Dadekian G, Etienne M, et al. Practicing internal medicine onboard the USNS COMFORT in the aftermath of the Haitian earthquake. Ann Intern Med 2010;152(11):733–7.
25. Vanholder R, Gibney N, Luyckx VA, et al. Renal disaster relief task force . Renal disaster relief task force in Haiti earthquake. Lancet 2010;375(9721):1162–3.
26. Haag R, Hembree-Bey RB, Mondiello M, et al. Infection prevention at a medical needs shelter for hurricane evacuees. Am J Infect Control 2013;41(6):S3.
27. Chew L, Ramdas KN. Caught in the storm: the impact of natural disasters on women. San Francisco (CA): The Global Fund for Women; 2005. Available at: http://www.globalfundforwomen.org/storage/images/stories/downloads/disaster-report.pdf. Accessed December 4, 2018.
28. Goodman A, Black L, Briggs S. Obstetrical care and women's health in the aftermath of disasters: the first 14 days after the 2010 Haitian earthquake. Am J Disaster Med 2014;9:59–65.
29. Oxford CM, Ludmir J. Trauma in pregnancy. Clin Obstet Gynecol 2009;52(4): 611–29.
30. McKinney P, Volkert P, Kaufman J. Fatal swine influenza pneumonia occurring during late pregnancy. Arch Intern Med 1990;150:213–5.
31. Kodali BS, Chandrasekhar S, Bulich LN, et al. Airway changes during labor and delivery. Anesthesiology 2008;108:357–62.
32. Elkus R, Popovich J. Respiratory physiology in pregnancy. Clin Chest Med 1992; 13:555–65.
33. Archer GW, Marx GF. Arterial oxygen tension during apnoea in parturient women. Br J Anaesth 1974;46:358–60.
34. Mabie WC, DiSessa TG, Crocker LG, et al. A longitudinal study of cardiac output in normal human pregnancy. Am J Obstet Gynecol 1994;170:849–56.
35. Konje JC, Kaufmann P, Bell SC, et al. A longitudinal study of quantitative uterine blood flow with the use of color power angiography in appropriate for gestational age pregnancies. Am J Obstet Gynecol 2001;185:608–13.
36. Kinsella SM, Lohmann G. Supine hypotensive syndrome. Obstet Gynecol 1994; 83:774–88.
37. Lederman MM. Cell-mediated immunity and pregnancy. Chest 1984;86:6S–9S.
38. Priddy KD. Immunologic adaptations during pregnancy. J Obstet Gynecol Neonatal Nurs 1997;26:388–94.
39. Lapinsky SE. Pregnancy joins the hit list. Crit Care Med 2012;40:1679–80.
40. Mattox KL, Goetzl L. Trauma in pregnancy. Crit Care Med 2005;33:385–9.
41. Pearlman MD, Tintinalli JE, Lorenz RP. Blunt trauma during pregnancy. N Engl J Med 1990;323:1609–13.

42. Hill C, Pickinpaugh J. Trauma and surgical emergencies in the obstetric patient. Surg Clin North Am 2008;88:421–40.

43. Ratnapalan S, Bentur Y, Koren G. Doctor, will that x-ray harm my unborn child? CMAJ 2008;179:1293–6.

44. American College of Obstetricians and Gynecologists' Committee on Obstetric Practice. Committee opinion No. 656: guidelines for diagnostic imaging during pregnancy and lactation. Obstet Gynecol 2016;127:e75–80.

45. Lowe SA. Diagnostic radiography in pregnancy: risks and reality. Aust N Z J Obstet Gynaecol 2004;44:191–6.

46. Assali NS. Dynamics of the uteroplacental circulation in health and disease. Am J Perinatol 1989;6:105–9.

47. Federal Drug Agency. FDA Drug Safety Communication: FDA review results in new warnings about using general anesthetics and sedation drugs in young children and pregnant women 2016. Available at: https://www.fda.gov/drugs/drugsafety/ucm532356.htm. Accessed December 4, 2018.

48. Aoyama K, Seaward PG, Lapinsky SE. Fetal outcome in the critically ill pregnant woman. Crit Care 2014;18:307.

49. Pollock W, Rose L, Dennis CL. Pregnant and postpartum admissions to the intensive care unit: a systematic review. Intensive Care Med 2010;36:1465–74.

50. Guntupalli KK, Hall N, Karnad DR, et al. Critical illness in pregnancy: part I: an approach to a pregnant patient in the ICU and common obstetric disorders. Chest 2015;148:1093–110.

51. Weinstein L. Syndrome of hemolysis, elevated liver enzymes, and low platelet count: a severe consequence of hypertension in pregnancy. Am J Obstet Gynecol 1982;142:159–67.

52. World Health Organization. WHO recommendations for Prevention and treatment of pre-eclampsia and eclampsia 2011. Available at: apps.who.int/iris/bitstream/handle/10665/44703/9789241548335_eng.pdf. Accessed December 5, 2018.

53. WOMAN Trial Collaborators. Effect of early tranexamic acid administration on mortality, hysterectomy, and other morbidities in women with post-partum haemorrhage (WOMAN): an international, randomised, double-blind, placebo-controlled trial. Lancet 2017;389:2105–16.

54. Lapinsky SE, Rojas-Suarez JA, Crozier TM, et al. Mechanical ventilation in critically-ill pregnant women: a case series. Int J Obstet Anesth 2015;24:323–8.

55. Hung CY, Hu HC, Chiu LC, et al. Maternal and Neonatal outcomes of respiratory failure during pregnancy. J Formos Med Assoc 2018;117:413–20.

56. Daniels K, Oakeson AM, Hilton G. Steps toward a national disaster plan for obstetrics. Obstet Gynecol 2014;124:154–8.

57. The International Federation of Gynecology and Obstetrics. Global library of women's medicine. Available at: http://www.glowm.com/contents. Accessed December 5, 2018.

58. Gray L, MacDonald C. Morbid obesity in disasters: bringing the "Conspicuously invisible" into focus. Int J Environ Res Public Health 2016;13:e75S–86S.

59. Geiling J. Critical care of the morbidly obese in disaster. Crit Care Clin 2010;26:703–14.

60. Institute of Medicine (US) Committee on guidance for establishing standards of care for use in disaster situations. In: Altevogt BM, Stroud C, Hanson SL, et al, editors. Guidance for establishing crisis standards of care for use in disaster situations: a letter report. Washington (DC): National Academies Press (US); 2009. Available at: https://www.ncbi.nlm.nih.gov/books/NBK219958/.

61. Biddinger PD, Cadigan RO, Auerbach BS, et al. On linkages: using exercises to identify systems-level preparedness challenges. Public Health Rep 2008;123(1): 96–101.
62. Sheridan R, Weber J, Prelack K, et al. Early burn center transfer shortens the length of hospitalization and reduces complications in children with serious burn injuries. J burn Care Rehabil 1999;20(5):347–50.
63. Biddison LD, Berkowitz KA, Courtney B, et al. Ethical considerations: care of the critically ill and injured during pandemics and disasters: CHEST consensus statement. Chest 2014;146(4 Suppl):e145S–55S.
64. Christian MD, Sprung CL, King MA, et al. Triage: care of the critically ill and injured during pandemics and disasters: CHEST consensus statement. Chest 2014;146(4 Suppl):e61S–74S.

Principles and Practices of Establishing a Hospital-Based Ebola Treatment Unit

Peter Kiiza, MBChB, DTM&H[a], Neill K.J. Adhikari, Msc[a,b,c],
Sarah Mullin, BSc(candidate)[a], Koren Teo, BScPHM, MHSc[d],
Robert A. Fowler, MS (Epi)[a,b,c],*

KEYWORDS

- Ebola • Outbreak • Treatment

KEY POINTS

- Hospital-based high-level pathogen and Ebola treatment practices should be established before there are suspected patients or an outbreak.
- Training a multidisciplinary team of health care workers in infection prevention and control and clinical management of patients with high-level pathogens, including Ebola, can increase staff confidence, reduce nosocomial infections, improve case detection, ensure safe waste management practices, and allow for standardized clinical care.
- Establishment of hospital-based Ebola treatment units facilitates care of patients with both Ebola-specific and nonspecific illness, leverages existent infrastructure and human resource capacity, and enables rapid adaptation to meet local demands.
- Interdisciplinary teams in disparately resourced settings should forge collaborations that strengthen research platforms, with the aim of pushing the boundaries of Ebola clinical care, diagnostics, vaccines, and therapeutics.

INTRODUCTION

The 2014 to 2016 West African Ebola virus disease (EVD) outbreak offered invaluable lessons to countries and provided impetus for health system preparedness.[1] Although a plethora of literature describing establishment of treatment units (ETU) for EVD

Competing Interests: None.
[a] Sunnybrook Research Institute, Sunnybrook Hospital, 2075 Bayview Avenue, Toronto, Ontario M4N 3M5, Canada; [b] Institute for Health Policy, Management and Evaluation, Dalla Lana School of Public Health, University of Toronto, Toronto, Ontario, Canada; [c] Interdepartmental Division of Critical Care Medicine, University of Toronto, Toronto, Ontario, Canada; [d] Canadian Forces Health Services Group, Toronto, 10 Yukon Ln, North York, Ontario M3K 0A1, Canada
* Corresponding author. 2075 Bayview Avenue, Room D478, Toronto, Ontario M4N 3M5, Canada.
E-mail address: Rob.fowler@sunnybrook.ca

patients in resource-rich settings exists,[1–11] literature outlining shared opportunities for hospital-based ETUs in high-income and resource-limited settings is scant.

On August 1, 2018, the World Health Organization (WHO) was notified of a swiftly unfolding EVD outbreak in North Kivu province, Democratic Republic of Congo (DRC).[12] As of July 21, 2019, 2592 confirmed and probable cases and 1743 deaths have been reported, with a case-fatality ratio (CFR) of 67%.[12] Since 1976, DRC has had 10 EVD outbreaks, with the current being the largest and most complex.[13]

Numerous factors are impeding efforts by DRC's Ministry of Health and partners to control the second deadliest EVD outbreak in history: armed conflicts, community distrust, and a reluctance to adopt recommended health precautions. Although the current outbreak remains centered in DRC, WHO performs regular risk assessments, given the concern for expansion of the outbreak and spread to other countries.[14]

HISTORICAL CARE AND ISOLATION OF PATIENTS WITH EBOLA

Since the 1960s, special isolation facilities have been built[1] to manage patients with highly infectious disease (eg, EVD, Marburg virus disease, and Lassa fever). However, the West African outbreak, unmatched in magnitude, longevity, and transmission dynamics, outstripped previously known containment measures,[1] requiring countries to reassess their capacities in managing highly infectious pathogens.[2] During the West African outbreak, isolation facilities differed in both design and care delivery. In resource-rich settings (Europe and United States), biocontainment units and modified intensive care units were used[1,3–11]; in West Africa, there were ETUs to assess and treat confirmed and suspect cases, and Ebola holding units (EHUs) positioned in hospitals to handle suspect cases before referral to ETUs.[2] Irrespective of the resources available or facility model chosen, a set of core principles should guide creation of ETUs, with requisite infection prevention and control (IPC) standards.[1–11]

This review describes principles and practices of establishing a hospital-based ETU and explores shared opportunities for disparately resourced settings. Lessons are drawn from published literature on ETUs and EHUs from resource-limited settings, and from hospitals that assessed suspected Ebola patients and biocontainment units in resource-rich settings during the 2014 to 2016 EVD outbreak.[1–11,15–20]

RATIONALE FOR ESTABLISHING A HOSPITAL-BASED EBOLA TREATMENT UNIT

With EVD and other high-risk pathogen-related illnesses occurring more frequently, health care workers (HCWs) and patients are increasingly at risk of outbreaks and subsequent nosocomial amplification.[15] WHO estimates that HCWs were 20 times more likely to become infected than the general population during the 2014 to 2016 EVD outbreak.[16]

Despite the current EVD outbreak ravaging DRC,[12] the risk for international spread is heightened given armed conflict and population migration.[14] Given the ease of travel by air in addition to land, nearby and all health systems should maintain preparedness to mitigate the risk of outbreaks. Practicing optimal IPC in all health settings will help to prevent the spread of all transmissible pathogens, not just Ebola.

CLINICAL PRESENTATION OF EBOLA

EVD often manifests initially with nonspecific symptoms and signs, fever, asthenia, myalgias, and anorexia, and progresses to a gastrointestinal clinical syndrome with vomiting, diarrhea, and subsequently, intravascular volume depletion, electrolyte imbalance, and organ dysfunction that requires acute or intensive supportive care.[17–20] Data from WHO estimated that the overall CFR during the West African outbreak was lower among patients admitted to hospitals (CFR 61%, 95% confidence interval [CI] 59%–62%) versus those not admitted (CFR 88%, 95% CI 86%–90%),[18] and even lower when supportive and critical care was introduced.[19] Thus, establishment of a hospital-based ETU offers patients timely access to basic supportive care and intensive care as required.

KEY PRINCIPLES AND PRACTICES FOR ESTABLISHING A HOSPITAL-BASED ESTABLISHMENT OF TREATMENT UNITS

These descriptions for setting up hospital-based ETUs could reasonably be extrapolated to other infectious diseases like Lassa or Marburg virus disease. Importantly, these recommendations should work within a framework of a resilient health system,[21] using existing local resources to strengthen immediate and long-term institutional capacity while being responsive and scalable to local epidemiology and evolving as research suggests ways to improve patient care.

Coordination and Operationalization of the Establishment of Treatment Units

Leadership and coordination
Hospital management of an EVD patient requires a multidisciplinary team from clinical care, IPC, environmental engineering, and administrative and nonhospital staff (such as provincial/state personnel).[4] An incident command structure with predefined roles for the diverse professions and departments involved should be formulated.[4]

Clinicians or hospital personnel with leadership experience managing high-risk pathogens are likely best suited to maintain and coordinate ETU preparedness and activities. Clinical teams and areas that will function as ETUs should adopt regularly practiced and standardized protocols to quickly operationalize patient management should a suspect case present.[1,18,22] A communication strategy with accepted codes of conduct when engaging the public should be stipulated.[3] Models of coordination structures can be drawn from facilities with experience of handling Ebola patients.[4] HCWs likely to encounter high-risk pathogens should have the opportunity for appropriate vaccinations, for example, with rVSV-ZEBOV vaccine,[23] despite lack of licensing.

Ambulance and transportation services
Where applicable, ETUs should collaborate with prehospital infrastructure (eg, ambulances) to ensure safe transportation of suspect and confirmed patients, referencing guidelines from experienced-technical organizations.[11,24–26]

Safe handling and transportation of a potentially infectious patient require significant expertise and practice among the team (eg, driver, supervisor, clinician, and IPC specialist) and collaboration with multiple partners (law enforcement and public health agencies, other hospitals, and transportation authorities).[3,23] Strict IPC precautions should be adhered to while transporting a potentially infectious patient, for example, a compartmentalized ambulance that separates driver and patient areas, personal protective equipment (PPE) commensurate to risk, and management of infectious spills according to established guidelines.[11,23–27]

Interdisciplinary teams
The formulation of an interprofessional team typically includes HCWs from emergency care, critical care, infectious diseases, IPC, pharmacy, laboratory, radiology, nutrition, social work, and security.[5,6] Standby medical expertise from pediatrics, anesthesia, obstetrics, nephrology, ophthalmology, and psychiatry should exist.

Volunteers from outside the hospital who have experience in high-risk pathogen treatment should be used in situations wherein staff are unable to join the ETU team.[3,7] In settings with chronic-skilled HCW shortages, task shifting should be considered, after appropriate training. This step is especially helpful when a rapid surge in patients overwhelms local health workforce capacity.[22]

Patient care pathway

Hospitals should define their own care pathways for patients with a potential high-risk pathogen (**Fig. 1**). Such patients should be assessed according to the suspect case definition on clinical and epidemiologic grounds as per applicable recommendations.[23–26,28] HCWs screening patients should take a history of patient symptoms, exposure, and travel history to high-risk areas during the potential incubation period (eg, the past 21 days for Ebola).[23,24] The screening process should take place in a room that meets IPC standards, with a 1- to 2-m barrier between the HCW and patients; alcohol-based hand rub (preferred over chlorine) and surface disinfectant; and separate access for patients and HCWs (**Fig. 2**). PPE required while screening should be proportional to risk but should include "light PPE" (face shield or goggles, gloves, and potentially, boots, gown, and an apron).[25,27] Potentially infectious patients need counseling and information on their course of care (IPC measures; movement restrictions within their room; laboratory investigations; and initial bundle of care). Relevant local health authorities should be notified.[25,26,28] After triage and the initial plan of care, an interdisciplinary team should regularly reassess patients[24] guided by clinical evolution and laboratory investigations.

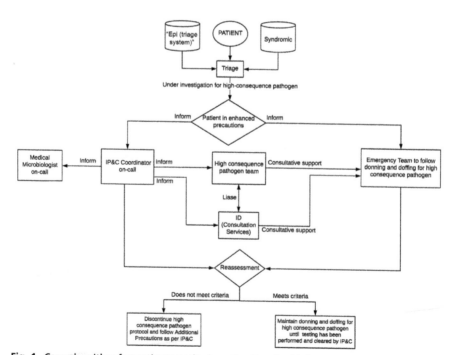

Fig. 1. Care algorithm for patients under investigation for high-consequence pathogen. ID, infectious diseases; IP&C, infection prevention and control. (*Courtesy of* From J Leis, MD, M.Sc, Toronto, ON, Canada.)

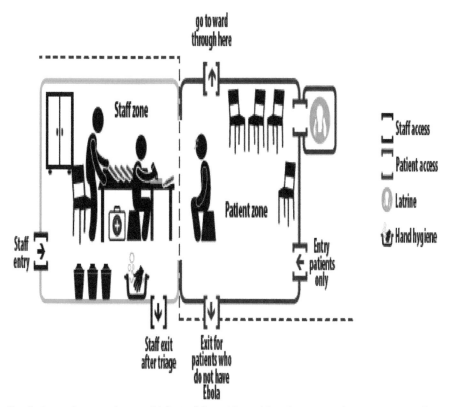

Fig. 2. Screening area layout. (*Adapted from* Manual for the care and management of patients in the Ebola care units/community care centres: interim emergency guidance. Geneva (Switzerland): World Health Organization; 2015. P. 5; with permission.)

Infrastructure: Design and Layout of the Hospital-Based Ebola Treatment Units

An appropriately located ETU is preferably physically separated from non-EVD care wards and easily accessible to ambulance drop-off points and to the pharmacy, medical equipment, and diagnostic testing.[5,26] The area should be sufficiently spacious to permit creation of multiple individual patient rooms to match a surge in cases.[5]

There is no universal design for the layout of an ETU; however, salient IPC principles should be followed during construction.[1–6,8,9] These IPC principles include secure entry and exit points; unidirectional flow of staff and patients with clear signage; donning and doffing areas adjacent to patient rooms; space for PPE storage[25]; clearly demarcated zones, that is, "green, low-risk zone" (donning area, visitors' area, and storage space, and so forth); and a "red, high-risk zone" (patient rooms and toilets, waste disposal area, and so forth).

Depending on the resources available, patient rooms (**Figs. 3** and **4**)[5] might allow for clinical documentation areas, patient relative(s) areas for direct, geographically separated, or technology-assisted communication (cameras, speakers, microphones), and separate point-of-care testing (to minimize transportation of infectious specimens). Rooms that can accommodate life-support equipment (oxygen systems, dialysis machines, ventilators, infusion pumps, and patient monitors), portable radiology and ultrasound machines[4–6,26] are required for critically ill patients. The design and operation of ETUs can be guided by published guidelines.[3,11,23,25,26]

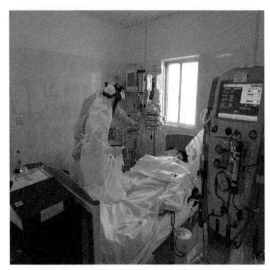

Fig. 3. An Ebola treatment facility, Goderich, Sierra Leone, February 2015. (*From* Leligdowicz A, Fischer WA, Uyeki TM, et al. Ebola virus disease and critical illness. Crit Care 2016; 20: 2.)

Logistics, Supplies, and Equipment

ETUs will have unique supply chains but should be aligned to existing supply chains whenever feasible[7] to ensure a consistent supply, avoid unnecessary stockpiling of available medical supplies, and free up HCWs to concentrate on other hospital or ETU activities.

The quantity and supplies required to run an ETU should be planned in advance and should include training materials and consumables and equipment, anticipating a

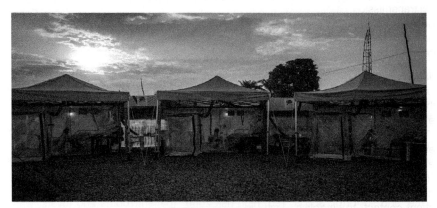

Fig. 4. Biosecure emergency care unit for outbreaks (CUBE). At the Alliance for International Medical Action's (ALIMA) Ebola Treatment Center in Beni, in the DRC's North Kivu Province, health workers care for patients infected with Ebola within ALIMA's innovative CUBE. The CUBE is a biosecure emergency care unit for outbreaks of highly infectious diseases, which allows HCWs to monitor the patient, check their vital signs, and administer certain treatments and care from the exterior, without having to wear full PPE. Family members can also safely talk with and see the patient throughout the course of treatment, thanks to the CUBE's transparent walls. This improves the treatment experience for the patient and their family. (Three biosecure emergency care units, known as the CUBE, are seen here at ALIMA's [The Alliance for International Medical Action] Ebola Treatment Center in Beni, in the Democratic Republic of the Congo. Photo: John Wessels/ALIMA.)

2-week length of stay per patient with EVD.[29] Advance assurance of a reliable supply chain, particularly for PPE, is essential given that an unanticipated surge of patients may overwhelm any local stockpile. Logistics personnel may use the WHO list of essential medicines and devices needed for EVD care[30,31] and tools to estimate the required quantity of PPE stock.[29]

Surveillance, Laboratory, Screening, and Triage at the Establishment of Treatment Units

Hospital-based surveillance for EVD is of paramount importance to the larger community. The ETU team should be part of strengthening this system.

A hospital-based disease surveillance system presumes that HCWs have been trained in detecting and responding to high-consequence transmissible diseases and appreciate that public health agencies must be notified.[28]

Electronic surveillance systems and medical records to augment widely available paper-based data systems facilitate communication between the red and green zones.[7] Standard case report forms should be available, with electronic copies on platforms such as mobile phones or tablets.

Screening

Regions with active EVD transmission and those areas at increased risk of receiving suspect cases should train hospital staff in the application of the national case definition.[23] Case definitions that evolve with outbreak epidemiology[23,28] should be reflected in screening tools.[4,23] ETU staff should conduct screening of patients and staff at strategic hospital entry points[7,32] (see **Fig. 2**).

In regions with on-going EVD outbreaks, screening should happen at hospital entry points and on inpatient wards. Of note, some patients may screen negative for EVD at triage, because no case definition is 100% sensitive, but later test positive on non-EVD wards.[33] Delay or absence of in-patient screening facilitates the potential for nosocomial transmission. Staff should have a high index of suspicion during interoutbreak periods and be able to apply the nonoutbreak case definitions.[23] HCW safety is a cornerstone of any outbreak; therefore, ETU staff needs periodic retraining on the screening process,[23,24] including daily self-screening assessments.

Triage

During outbreaks, HCWs should screen patients for signs and symptoms of EVD, while also sorting them according to illness severity.[34] The sickest patients should be triaged and prioritized for acute or emergency care.[34,35]

The use of validated triage tools to guide rapid identification and treatment of emergency signs and symptoms should be used. HCWs in resource-limited settings should be trained in the application of triage tools.[35–37]

In areas with Ebola transmission, modifications in the screening/triage process are often warranted, that is, use of only visual signs, as opposed to vital signs that require patient contact, to establish whether a patient needs urgent treatment. Most emergency signs (difficulty in breathing, altered level of consciousness, seizures, bleeding) can be assessed visually and augmented with a brief history. Suspect patients with emergency signs require urgent response by teams in full PPE working in appropriate environments.[24,34]

Laboratory

Early clinical diagnosis of EVD is challenging because many symptoms and signs are nonspecific.[17] The ability to perform rapid diagnostic tests enables early case detection and monitoring of disease progression and guides timing of patient discharge.[38]

Molecular testing using reverse transcription polymerase chain reaction (RT-PCR) on whole blood samples is the recommended confirmatory EVD test in live patients.[23,39] Each jurisdiction should have guidance for timely laboratory diagnosis at a reference laboratory or local laboratories that can run nucleic acid tests (eg, GeneXpert).[39] Rapid antigen tests, although imperfectly sensitive, might be considered for screening suspect patients[24,26,38-40] where molecular testing is unavailable.

Point-of-care tests, including blood counts, biochemistry, liver function and coagulation tests, and rapid tests for malaria and pregnancy, are recommended.[6] These tests collectively enable appreciation and treatment of underlying physiologic derangements and important concomitant conditions.[7] Traditional blood cultures or novel molecular diagnostics for bacterial infections may not be commonly available in all settings but are crucial to identify alternative foci of infection for patients with EVD.

Risk of collection and transportation of EVD samples can be mitigated through adherence to IPC precautions,[24-26] staff training, and triple packaging systems.[39,40] Protocols for sample collection and transportation from the Centers for Disease Control and Prevention, WHO, and other national public health laboratory are available for adaptation.[23-26]

Clinical Care

The clinical management of EVD patients over prior and recent outbreaks has witnessed remarkable progress, with several experienced organizations and clinical personnel championing evidence-based guidelines.[41,42] Literature detailing protocols for the clinical care of EVD patients is available.[23-26,32,40-43]

A recent systematic review[44] of anti-Ebola virus therapies revealed that less than 5% of EVD patients have been enrolled in studies of these treatments, with inferences limited by nonrandomized study designs. The only randomized controlled trial published to date enrolled 72 patients and compared the monoclonal antibody ZMapp to standard care (mortality, 22% vs 37%; 95% CI for risk difference, 36%–7%). Studies of convalescent plasma, interferon-β-1a, favipiravir, brincidofovir, artesunate-amodiaquine, and TKM-130803 were associated with at least moderate risk of bias limiting inferences on effectiveness. An ongoing clinical trial in the DRC is evaluating 3 anti-Ebola monoclonal antibodies (mAb114, ZMapp, and REGN3470-3471-3479), and an antiviral drug (remdesivir).[39,41]

Just less than half (41%) of EVD patients treated in Europe and the United States during the 2014 to 2016 outbreak developed severe illness requiring intensive care, including respiratory support with noninvasive or invasive ventilation; cardiovascular support with central venous and arterial catheterization, cardiopulmonary resuscitation, or intravenous vasoactive medications; or some form of dialysis.[4-8,17-20,42] As resource-limited settings gain experience with EVD, some aspects of critical care should be implemented.[22]

Clinical care protocols and guidelines
Previous successful implementation and adaptation of checklists/guidelines for the management of sepsis, surgical complications, and ventilation and similar issues have reduced mortality and morbidity in various resource settings.[22] A recent evidence-based guideline[42] detailed 8 key recommendations for supportive care for patients with EVD in resource-limited settings. Global adoption of these guidelines should create an environment of accountability and uniformity in quality of care.

Palliative care
All patients should ideally have access to end-of-life care that focuses on preventing and treating common symptoms, such as pain and breathlessness. Protocols for end-

of-life care that incorporate local norms and culture and views from survivors where possible should be developed.[17,45]

Staffing ratio and patient monitoring

A staffing model should consider tiered needs, with a "rapid response team" to handle the first 1 to 2 patients and define patient thresholds for engaging additional staff.[7]

In resource-limited settings, evidence-based guidelines strongly recommend an ETU staffing ratio of 1 clinician to 4 patients, with at least 3 patient assessments per day[42] to enable timely appreciation of clinical changes and clinician response.

In resource-rich settings, the US National Institutes of Health recommends a minimum number of personnel to effectively manage a severely ill patient for 1 week, expressed per 8-hour shift, as 2 nurses (6 per day), 1 to 2 physicians (3–4 per day), and 1 PPE adherence monitor (3 per day).[10]

Clinical monitoring and documentation should include vital signs, symptoms, volume assessment, laboratory parameters, and overall clinical status.[42] Early warning scores for clinical deterioration may be considered.[24,42] Case report forms are available from WHO and can be adapted to the local context.[46]

Nutritional support

Nutritional support should be part of routine care.[24] Cautious supplementary enteral rehydration and feeding should be encouraged in patients with inadequate intake secondary to anorexia, vomiting, diarrhea, odynophagia, or reduced level of consciousness.[47] In children, nutritional assessments should be conducted before initiating fluid resuscitation and nutrition.[47] WHO recommends that breast milk from infected mothers should not be given to uninfected or infected babies[24]; supplemental nutritional recommendations in the context of EVD are available for children.[47]

Communication and psychological support

A communications strategy to educate patients, patients' families and friends, and HCWs about EVD presentation, prevention, and treatments complements the acute care response.[39] Messages should be simple and transparent, should acknowledge knowledge gaps, and should be tailored to perceived staff and patient concerns. Staff and their families should have access to psychological support.[7,23]

Care for special patient categories

The care for pregnant women, infants and young children (without caretakers), and surgical patients can be extremely challenging. Modifications are needed in the operations of an ETU; for example, creation of mother-baby care units, stocking infant nutrition, potential employment of Ebola survivors as caretakers of ill babies, and dedicated operating rooms for birthing and cesarean sections are just a few of the important considerations. Protocols detailing holistic care of mothers, babies, and families should be in place.[9,24,48,49]

Discharge criteria and support care for survivors

Discharge of a convalescent Ebola patient is generally based on the following principles: clinical improvement (symptom-free or no symptoms of viral shedding, ie, diarrhea, vomiting, or bleeding), ability to perform activities of daily living, and 1 or 2 negative serum Ebola RT-PCR tests.[23,24] Guidelines for the discharge, follow-up, and community reintegration of survivors are available.[23–25,40]

Clinical Data Management

There is limited guidance for clinical documentation, data capture tools, and data transfer methods from patient wards during outbreaks in resource-limited settings.

Before the West African outbreak, a survey[50] was used to explore optimal documentation and data transfer methods from EVD wards. In settings with no electricity, most experts recommended to have 1 clinician review patients as another takes notes, with the second clinician dictating findings to another HCW outside the red zone. Where electricity is available, recommendations are to use tablets, smartphones, or laptops in the red zone, with data transmission over a local wireless or wired network.

Infection Prevention and Control

HCWs providing EVD care should observe both standard and transmission-based precautions.[24]

Standard and contact precautions, including hand and respiratory hygiene, PPE use, prevention of needle stick injuries, environmental cleaning and disinfection, and waste management, are an essential component in reducing the risk of transmission of EVD.[24] Although standard and contact precautions are the mainstay of IPC, droplet precautions are often also used in the care of patients with EVD. Airborne-based precautions are appropriate when there is a concern of aerosol-generating procedures or conditions.[23]

Because proper hand washing is a key to preventing transmission of the virus,[23] hand-washing facilities and wall charts (highlighting hand-washing steps) should be provided in all patient care areas. Alcohol-based liquids or gels should be used to sanitize not-visibly soiled hands, whereas soap and water or chlorine solution (0.05% concentration) is recommended for more soiled hands.[23]

Personal protective equipment

A WHO expert panel[27] strongly recommended the following PPE components: face shield/goggles, fluid-resistant medical/surgical mask with structured noncollapsing designs (eg, duckbill/cup shape), N-95 respirators (for aerosol generating procedures), 2 pairs of gloves (ideally different colors and preferably nitrile over latex gloves), impermeable coverall/gown, waterproof apron, reusable heavy duty gloves (for cleaning), rubber gumboots, and a head cover. Approved specifications for the different PPE components are available in technical documents.[25,27] The evidence base validating the safest sequence for PPE donning and doffing is of low quality.[51] Although donning and doffing practices might differ across institutions, technical organizations have issued comprehensive guidance on PPE use.[25,26] Large posters detailing donning and doffing steps, using a buddy system, should be displayed (**Fig. S1**A, B).[52]

Cleaning, disinfection, and waste management

Care of EVD patients can generate enormous amounts of infectious waste (up to 10 L of liquid waste and 40 large bags/patient/d).[6] Segregation, transportation, and disposal of such waste present huge challenges. ETUs could install autoclaves or steam sterilizers to sterilize waste onsite rather than contracting commercial vendors, who would require appropriate training. Construction of underground pits or incinerators to dispose of waste is appropriate in resource-limited settings.[6,23] Planning for waste management practices that maximize community safety should engage clinicians, IPC and environmental specialists, and security personnel.[3]

Floors, walls, and medical equipment should be cleaned and disinfected at least once daily or whenever soiled.[24,25] Extreme care should be taken while handling, cleaning, and disinfecting soiled equipment; in addition to full PPE, heavy gloves and aprons should be used.[27]

A list of registered hospital disinfectants effective against Ebola virus is available.[25] HCWs should be trained on the preparation and applications of different bleaching agents (chlorine concentrations, 0.5% and 0.05%, and alcohol).[23]

Staff should be trained on the standard operating procedures to handle, segregate, clean, disinfect, or dispose of medical waste and equipment and the distinction between reusable and non-reusable items. Details of these procedures are available.[24,25]

Training and Quality Improvement Activities

The room for HCW error in adhering to established IPC practices while caring for Ebola patients is small because of the risk of nosocomial transmission. Regular HCW training in EVD care and PPE use will allay anxiety and reduce the risk of error[10] and should be mandated to ensure competency.[6] Training should not only emphasize donning and doffing PPE but also the practice of simulated care tasks while in PPE. Training methods might include didactic, on-line, and hands-on sessions, and low- or high-fidelity simulations.[23–26,40]

Simulation sessions covering all aspects of EVD care should involve all ETU staff and might include examples of routine or challenging situations, such as extraction of collapsed HCWs from patient wards, multiple simultaneous suspect patient admissions, resuscitation of critically ill patients, and medical procedures, such as placing intravenous or intraosseous catheters.[6]

Research

As the improvement of patient care remains a critical aspect of an outbreak response, it is imperative for stakeholders to support processes that enhance implementation of observational and interventional studies before, during, and after outbreaks.[17,22]

There are frequent delays in initiating outbreak-focused studies, including protocol development; application, review and submission to research ethics boards, data sharing agreements, contracts, and financial agreements.[15] Teams should identify anticipated bottlenecks and engage their respective stakeholders in advance. Pre-approved research protocols prior to outbreaks, centralized ethics committees, common data elements and data collection tools, and the experience of seasoned clinicians and established clinical research groups[13,15] may improve research efficiency during an outbreak.

SUMMARY

With an increasing frequency of infectious disease outbreaks worldwide and increased ease of global travel, the establishment of context-appropriate robust clinical care for patients with high-consequence and transmissible pathogens is relevant to all health systems. Establishing hospital-based ETUs is 1 step toward the improvement of patient care. However, establishing an ETU in environments unfamiliar with the illness requires interdisciplinary and interprofessional coordination and commitment; advance planning and HCW training; and a culture of flexibility that supports continuous preparedness and evaluation activities. Incorporating lessons learned from recent and current outbreaks and the knowledge of improved patient outcomes with improved patient care gives us the best chance at treating patients, keeping HCWs safe, and minimizing the risk for disease transmission in hospitals.

SUPPLEMENTARY DATA

Supplementary data related to this article can be found online at https://doi.org/10.1016/j.ccc.2019.06.011.

REFERENCES

1. Kortepeter MG, Kwon EH, Hewlett AL, et al. Containment care units for managing patients with highly hazardous infectious diseases: a concept whose time has come. J Infect Dis 2016;214:S137–41.
2. Johnson O, Youkee D, Brown CS, et al. Ebola holding units at government hospitals in Sierra Leone: evidence for a flexible and effective model for safe isolation, early treatment initiation, hospital safety and health system functioning. BMJ Glob Health 2016;1(1):e000030.
3. Smith PW, Boulter KC, Hewlett AL, et al. Planning and response to Ebola virus disease: an integrated approach. Am J Infect Control 2015;43:441–6.
4. Haverkort JJ, Minderhoud AL, Wind JD, et al. Hospital preparedness for viral hemorrhagic fever patients and experience gained from admission of an Ebola patient. Emerg Infect Dis 2016;22(2):184–91.
5. Leligdowicz A, Fischer WA, Uyeki TM, et al. Ebola virus disease and critical illness. Crit Care 2016;20:217.
6. Garibaldi BT, Chertow DS. High-containment pathogen preparation in the intensive care unit. Infect Dis Clin North Am 2017;31(3):561–76.
7. Grein JD, Murthy AR. Preparing a hospital for Ebola virus disease: a review of lessons learned. Curr Treat Options Infect Dis 2016;8(4):237–50.
8. Martin D, Howard J, Agarwal B, et al. The UK critical care perspective. Br J Anaesth 2016;116(5):590–6.
9. DeBiasi RL, Song X, Cato K, et al. Preparedness, evaluation, and care of pediatric patients under investigation for Ebola virus disease: experience from a pediatric designated care facility. J Pediatric Infect Dis Soc 2015;5(1):68–75.
10. Decker BK, Sevransky JE, Barrett K, et al. Preparing for critical care services to patients with Ebola. Ann Intern Med 2014;161(11):831–2.
11. Bannister B, Puro V, Fusco FM, et al. Group EW framework for the design and operation of high-level isolation units: consensus of the European Network of Infectious Diseases. Lancet Infect Dis 2009;9:45–56.
12. WHO. Ebola situation reports. Available at: https://www.who.int/ebola/situation-reports/drc-2018/en/. Accessed July 23, 2019.
13. CDC. Outbreak chronology. Ebola virus disease. Available at: https://www.cdc.gov/vhf/ebola/history/chronology.html. Accessed April 25, 2018.
14. WHO. Ebola situation reports. Available at: https://apps.who.int/iris/bitstream/handle/10665/273640/SITREP_EVD_DRC_20180807-eng.pdf?ua=1. Accessed April 25, 2018.
15. Rishu AH, Marinoff N, Julien L, et al. Time required to initiate outbreak and pandemic observational research. J Crit Care 2017;40:7–10.
16. WHO. Ebola response roadmap situation report. 2014. Available at: http://apps.who.int/iris/bitstream/10665/133833/1/roadmapsitrep4_eng.pdf?ua=1. Accessed April 24, 2018.
17. Fowler RA, Fletcher T, Fischer WA 2nd, et al. Caring for critically ill patients with Ebola virus disease. Perspectives from West Africa. Am J Respir Crit Care Med 2014;190:733–7.
18. Rojek A, Horby P, Dunning J. Insights from clinical research completed during the West Africa Ebola virus disease epidemic. Lancet Infect Dis 2017;17(9):e280–92.
19. Langer M, Portella G, Finazzi S, et al. Intensive care support and clinical outcomes of patients with Ebola virus disease (EVD) in West Africa. Intensive Care Med 2018;44(8):1266–75.

20. Uyeki TM, Mehta AK, Davey RT Jr, et al, Working group of the U.S.–European Clinical Network on Clinical Management of Ebola Virus Disease Patients in the U.S. and Europe. Clinical management of Ebola virus disease in the United States and Europe. N Engl J Med 2016;374(7):636–46.

21. Kruk ME, Myers M, Varpilah ST, et al. What is a resilient health system? Lessons from Ebola. Lancet 2015;385:1910–2.

22. Kerry VB, Sayeed S. Leveraging opportunities for critical care in resource-limited settings. Glob Heart 2014;9(3):275.

23. WHO. Ebola key technical documents. 2017. Available at: https://www.who.int/ebola/22-5-17-Ebola-Key-technical-documents-EN.pdf?ua=1. Accessed April 26, 2019.

24. WHO. Clinical management of patients with viral haemorrhagic fever: a pocket guide for front-line health workers: interim emergency guidance for country adaptation. Available at: https://apps.who.int/iris/bitstream/handle/10665/205570/?sequence=1.

25. CDC. Ebola(ebola virus disease). For clinicians. Available at: https://www.cdc.gov/vhf/ebola/clinicians/index.html. Accessed February, 2019.

26. Ebola clinical care guidelines. A guide to clinicians in Canada. Available at: https://caep.ca/wpcontent/uploads/2016/03/ebola_clinical_care_guideline_english_201505.pdf. Accessed January 19, 2019.

27. WHO. PPE for use in a filovirus disease outbreak. Rapid advice guideline. 2016. Available at: https://apps.who.int/iris/bitstream/handle/10665/251426/9789241549721-eng.pdf?sequence=1. Accessed April, 2019.

28. WHO/CDC. Guidelines for integrated disease surveillance and response in the African Region: 1-398. 2010. Available at: https://www.cdc.gov/globalhealth/healthprotection/idsr/pdf/technicalguidelines/idsr-technical-guidelines-2nd-edition_2010_english.pdf.

29. CDC. Estimated personal protective equipment (PPE) needed for healthcare facilities. Available at: https://www.cdc.gov/vhf/ebola/healthcare-us/ppe/calculator.html. Accessed February 2, 2019.

30. WHO list of essential medicines necessary to treat Ebola cases. Available at: https://www.who.int/csr/resources/publications/ebola/ebola-medicines/en/. Accessed January 18, 2019.

31. WHO. WHO list medical devices for Ebola care. 2014. Available at: https://www.who.int/medical_devices/meddev_list_ebola_25nov_en.pdf?ua=1. Accessed January 18, 2019.

32. WHO. Manual for the care and management of patients in the Ebola care units/community care centres: interim emergency guidance. 2015. Available at: https://apps.who.int/iris/bitstream/handle/10665/149781/WHO_EVD_Manual_ECU_15.1_eng.pdf;jsessionid=098909AD6D93077A36F2017C35329F0D?sequence=1. Accessed May 1, 2019.

33. Dunn AC, Walker TA, Redd J, et al. Nosocomial transmission of Ebola virus disease on pediatric and maternity wards: Bombali and Tonkolili, Sierra Leone, 2014. Am J Infect Control 2016;44(3):269–72.

34. WHO. Quick check and emergency treatments for adolescents and adults 2011. Available at: http://www.who.int/influenza/patient_ care/clinical/IMAI_Wall_chart.pdf. Accessed January 19, 2019.

35. Cummings MJ, Wamala JF, Bakamutumaho B, et al. Vital signs: the first step in prevention and management of critical illness in resource-limited settings. Intensive Care Med 2016;42(9):1519.

36. Tamburlini G, Di Mario S, Maggi RS, et al. Evaluation of guidelines for emergency triage assessment and treatment in developing countries. Arch Dis Child 1999; 81(6):478–82.
37. WHO. Basic emergency care: approach to the acutely ill and injured 2018. Available at: https://www.who.int/emergencycare/publications/Basic-Emergency-Care/en/. Accessed May 05, 2019.
38. Broadhurst MJ, Brooks TJ, Pollock NR. Diagnosis of Ebola virus disease: past, present, and future. Clin Microbiol Rev 2016;29(4):773–93.
39. WHO. Ebola virus disease. Fact sheet. 2018. Available at: https://www.who.int/news-room/fact-sheets/detail/ebola-virus-disease. Accessed January 9, 2018.
40. Ebola virus infection-guidelines/BMJ best practice. Available at: https://bestpractice.bmj.com/topics/en-us/1210/guidelines. Accessed April 25, 2019.
41. Lamontagne F, Clément C, Kojan R, et al. The evolution of supportive care for Ebola virus disease. Lancet 2019;393(10172):620–1.
42. Lamontagne F, Fowler RA, Adhikari NK, et al. Evidence-based guidelines for supportive care of patients with Ebola virus disease. Lancet 2018;391(10121):700–8.
43. Clément C, Adhikari NK, Lamontagne F. Evidence-based clinical management of Ebola virus disease and epidemic viral hemorrhagic fevers. Infect Dis Clin North Am 2019;33(1):247–64.
44. James SL, Adhikari NK, Henry YK, et al. Anti-Ebola therapy for patients with Ebola virus disease: a systematic review. BMC Infect Dis 2019;19:376.
45. Nouvet E, Kouyaté S, Bezanson K, et al. Preparing for the dying and 'dying in honor': Guineans' perceptions of palliative care in Ebola treatment centers. J Pain Symptom Manage 2018;56(6):e55–6.
46. WHO. Ebola case report forms for clinicians. 2018. Available at: https://www.who.int/csr/resources/publications/ebola/case-report-forms-for-clinicians/en/. Accessed February 2, 2019.
47. WHO/UNICEF/WFP. Interim guideline: nutritional care of children and adults with Ebola virus disease in treatment centres. Geneva (Switzerland): World Health Organization; 2014.
48. WHO. Interim guidance ebola virus disease in pregnancy: screening and management of Ebola cases, contacts and survivors. 2018. Available at: https://apps.who.int/iris/bitstream/handle/10665/184163/WHO_EVD_HSE_PED_15.1_eng.pdf?ua=1. Accessed January 19, 2019.
49. Badia JM, Rubio-Pérez I, Díaz JA, et al. Surgical protocol for confirmed or suspected cases of Ebola and other highly transmissible diseases. Cir Esp 2016; 94(1):11–5.
50. Bühler S, Roddy P, Nolte E, et al. Clinical documentation and data transfer from Ebola and Marburg virus disease wards in outbreak settings: health care workers' experiences and preferences. Viruses 2014;6(2):927–37.
51. Verbeek JH, Ijaz S, Mischke C, et al. Personal protective equipment for preventing highly infectious diseases due to exposure to contaminated body fluids in healthcare staff. Cochrane Database Syst Rev 2016;(4):CD011621.
52. WHO. How to put on and how to remove personal protective equipment-posters 2015. Available at: https://www.who.int/csr/resources/publications/ebola/ppe-steps/en/. Accessed May 5, 2019.

Battling Superstorm Sandy at Lenox Hill Hospital
When the Hospital Is Ground Zero

Maciej Walczyszyn, MD[a], Shalin Patel, MD[b], Maly Oron, MD[c],*,
Bushra Mina, MD, FCCM, FCCP[d]

KEYWORDS

- Superstorm Sandy • Disaster management • Emergency command center
- Hospital evacuation

KEY POINTS

- The severity and impact of natural disasters are always unpredictable.
- Hospitals may face a challenge in dealing with a substantial influx of transferred patients from evacuated hospitals.
- When large medical centers are incapacitated, support centers are crucial for maintaining patient care and safety with both immediate and long-term relief.

HYPOTHESIS

When large medical centers become debilitated, patient care needs to be distributed to other functional facilities. "Accommodations must be made for both a disaster-related surge in patients and the usual intake of patients with unrelated urgent medical and surgical needs."[1]

INTRODUCTION

Nicknamed "Superstorm Sandy," Sandy is regarded as one of the deadliest, most destructive, and costliest hurricanes of the 2012 Atlantic hurricane season. The storm struck New York City on October 29, 2012. The Centers for Disease Control and Prevention estimates 53 fatalities in New York State, of which 43 occurred in New York City.[2,3] The damage to New York City was estimated at 19 billion dollars. More than

---

Disclosure Statement: The authors have nothing to disclose.
[a] Pulmonary Critical Care Division, Flushing Hospital Medical Center, 4500 Parsons Boulevard, Flushing, NY 11355, USA; [b] Medstar Georgetown University Hospital/MedStar Montgomery Medical Center, 18101 Prince Philip Drive, Olney, MD 20832, USA; [c] Pulmonary Critical Care Division, Lenox Hill Hospital, Northwell Health, 100 East 77th Street, New York, NY 10075, USA; [d] Pulmonary Critical Care Fellowship, Lenox Hill Hospital, Northwell Health, 100 East 77th Street, New York, NY 10075, USA
* Corresponding author.
E-mail address: malyoron@gmail.com

Crit Care Clin 35 (2019) 711–715
https://doi.org/10.1016/j.ccc.2019.06.012
0749-0704/19/© 2019 Elsevier Inc. All rights reserved.

305 thousand housing units were either damaged or destroyed.[2] "Thousands were displaced from their homes, and 2 major hospitals required perilous evacuations even as the hurricane-force winds engulfed the metropolitan region."[4]

One of the support centers that responded was Lenox Hill Hospital (LHH), a 652-bed tertiary care center. LHH has 3 separate intensive care units, each having 12 dedicated beds and an additional 17 monitored step-down beds per unit. There are 8 full-time intensivists and 6 Critical Care fellows available 24 hours per day, 7 days a week.

METHODS

Relying on LHH's previous experience from Storm Irene, as well as the knowledge of current employees who worked during 9/11 in the St. Vincent Hospital response, emergency preparations at LHH began 4 days before the storm. Emergency Command Centers were activated. With a prestorm census of 397, the hospital rapidly discharged all those who could be safely released to other facilities or to their homes to increase capacity. A "stretch to flex up and restock the house" strategy was applied by consolidating patient floors to provide entirely vacant units. Having complete and available floors allowed for improved organization of staffing and patient placement once the patient volume started to arrive. Furthermore, previously unutilized units and office space were prepared for patient accommodation and care with appropriate bedding and equipment.

Emergency teams were assigned; plans for medications and supplies were implemented, and transfer protocols were activated.[5] North Shore–Long Island Jewish (LIJ) Health System delivered 50 beds with over-bed tables as well as all other requested equipment and supplies. LHH generally has a reserve of 26 invasive and 14 noninvasive ventilators. In preparation for Sandy, an additional 10 invasive and 5 noninvasive ventilators were rented, increasing the reserve by 37.5%. Additional intravenous fluids, as well as an increased stock of surgical instrument sets and portable oxygen cylinders, were brought in (Hurricane Sandy—After Action Report/Improvement Plan).

Most of the LHH departments placed their staff in "on-call alert," and employees that lived outside of Manhattan were asked to stay locally with friends or relatives in case their services were required. For those who could not find nearby lodging, arrangements were made within the hospital, turning one of the hospital's auditoriums into staff accommodations using air mattresses (Hurricane Sandy—After Action Report/Improvement Plan).

The hospital's physical plant was assessed 48 hours before hurricane landfall to ensure the proper function of power generators, steam service, municipal water service to the facility, availability of fuel supply for generators, and adequate protection of the oxygen storage system from the storm (Hurricane Sandy—After Action Report/Improvement Plan).

RESULTS

On the day of the storm, early Monday morning of October 29, 2012, LHH Command Center was unexpectedly notified by the Center of Emergency Medical Services that the New York University (NYU) Langone Medical Center was being emergently shut down because of backup generator failure, prompting the evacuation of hundreds of patients, including those from the hospital's intensive care units. The LHH admission coordination team and communication protocols were activated. A paper bed board was established in case of electrical problems. Transport, medical, surgical, and critical care teams were made available in the emergency department (ED) to accept patients.

Storm Irene taught us that there needed to be a "hard stop" to control transferred patients whereby LHH staff can perform their own triage. It was decided that each patient would go through the ED and that no direct transfers would take place except into the neonatal intensive care unit. After triage, patients would be distributed based on the severity of illness as well as bed and nursing availability. Triage allowed LHH doctors to reevaluate each patient after transfer for any possible decompensation. It provided for organized, steady, and accurate floor, bed, nurse, and physician team assignments.

LHH received a total of 102 evacuees from surrounding hospitals, with the bulk (86% of patients) coming from NYU Langone Medical Center. Sixty-two percent of the NYU patients were admitted between 3 and 6 AM, equaling 1 patient every 3 minutes. Most of the patients were admitted to the regional floors; however, a significant number required a higher level of care (**Fig. 1**). At that time, all patients were admitted to LHH physician teams with limited patient information owing to an inaccessible NYU electronic medical record system.[5] Individual residents were explicitly assigned to contact their NYU counterparts for patient information. The medical and surgical teams' diligent work during triage and admissions resulted in zero adverse events in the LHH relief efforts. Within 24 hours, the medical and surgical team censuses nearly doubled with NYU transfer patients; however, this was only the beginning.

In the first week after Sandy, the workload increased tremendously, as LHH staff primarily handled patient care. Because of the high volume of incoming patients and continued lack of functional facilities at NYU, a satellite office for credentialing was established. In the following days, 315 NYU physicians and licensed independent practitioners were given Disaster Emergency privileges at LHH; more than 700 NYU nurses were credentialed and oriented to LHH, and 160 NYU residents and fellows were added by the Office of Graduate Medical Education.[5]

After the storm, occupancy at LHH persisted from 99% to 107% with an average daily census of 493 to 550 patients. LHH transitioned to a 7-d/wk operation performing operative elective procedures on Saturdays and Sundays.[5]

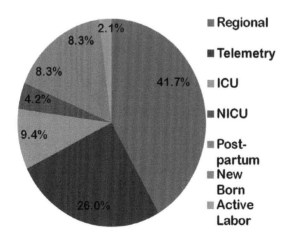

Fig. 1. Distribution of all transferred patients to LHH during the Sandy Superstorm. ICU, intensive care unit; NICU, neonatal intensive care unit.

INTERNAL MEDICINE

The Internal Medicine teams were supplemented with extra residents pulled from clinics and electives to be available to assist with the additional patient load. A plan for geographic floor coverage by residents was made to facilitate communication, especially in the case of a power outage. Most patients transferred from NYU arrived without medical records. Therefore, working directly with the NYU residents and hospitalists from Tisch Hospital, who came the next day, was crucial. The residents were given assumed privileges under the Graduate Medical Education affiliation agreement with NYU and, as in other departments, attending physicians had to obtain emergency privileges as well. A parallel service consisting of medical residents, students, and attendings was created to care for NYU patients on the general medical floors, making the workload more manageable despite the high census.

INTENSIVE CARE

Intensive care triage was performed in the ED on arrival of evacuated patients by LHH intensivist-led teams. Unlike the regional medical floors, where teams consisting of NYU physicians were caring for admitted NYU patients, the intensive care and step-down units remained under LHH care personnel only. These units routinely operate as closed units and remained as such after the storm, solely managed by LHH intensivists. In the first week following Storm Sandy, scheduled work hours were increased to allow the availability of a fellow on site at all times for critically ill patient management with a supervising intensivist. To accommodate the large flow of patients, 1 chief and 2 supervising respiratory therapists took 48-hour call shifts alternately during that period. Direct communication with the NYU health care staff was maintained, and upon discharge from ICU or telemetry, transfer summaries were provided for each patient.

PULMONARY

Similarly to the ED, the LHH pulmonary team fully assimilated their NYU counterparts. Two attending physicians and 2 fellows were emergently credentialed by the Medicine Board and seamlessly integrated into the bronchoscopy suite schedule. Cases were prioritized and rescheduled as needed to accommodate all procedures with ancillary support and cytologic evaluation as required. The Pulmonary consult services functioned independently; however, LHH pulmonary coverage was available for immediate assistance if the NYU staff was off-site.

SURGERY

The surgical teams were eventually integrated as well. Immediately after Sandy, the LHH residents were spread thinly between the LHH and the early credentialed NYU surgical attendings. It took approximately 2 weeks for the remainder of the NYU surgical staff to arrive at LHH, including residents, physician assistants, as well as nurses. Because of the lack of facilities and operating room times, most NYU patient surgeries were performed on weekends unless emergent. LHH residents were able to assist if cleared by the attending managing each case. This collaboration allowed for the full and safe care of all patients.

PATHOLOGY

The Pathology department expanded their frozen section coverage in the Anatomic Pathology (AP) laboratory from 5 to 7 days a week in order to accommodate the expanded operating room services. As expected, the number of surgical specimens in the AP laboratory increased significantly, particularly as NYU physicians began to admit patients to LHH, as did the number of tests in the clinical laboratory, requiring a limited amount of surgical specimens to be sent out to the Core Laboratory at North Shore–LIJ.

SUMMARY

The severity and impact of natural disasters are always unpredictable, and in the case of Hurricane Sandy, that was no exception. Although not suffering any significant physical or infrastructural damage because of the storm, LHH's most significant challenge was dealing with a substantial influx of transferred patients from evacuated hospitals. When large medical centers are incapacitated, support centers are crucial for maintaining patient care and safety with both immediate and long-term relief. The hospital's measures resulted in zero adverse events, indicating adequate preparation in all aspects, ranging from ensuring enough hospital beds were available as well as necessary supply, to assuring sufficient staffing of all departments. Once the initial threat of the storm settled, the key elements in maintaining large volume safe patient care were the integration of the disabled facility's (mainly NYU) personnel at all levels (nursing, residents, attendings, and so forth), maintaining open lines of communication, and continually reevaluating the quality of care. This task took not only organization but also experience from dealing with previous disasters. Some of the significant challenges included an increase in work hours and mental burden experienced by the staff as well as technical difficulties, such as medical records not transferred with patients arriving to LHH or adequate workspace to accommodate the visiting personnel. Future considerations to improve efficiency in similar occurrences should include implementing a designated disaster relief team for each large metropolitan area that coordinates intrahospital transfers, organizes communication of vital patient information, and expedites staff credentialing during emergency situations.

REFERENCES

1. Redlener I, Reilly MJ. Lessons from Sandy—preparing health systems for future disasters. N Engl J Med 2012;13:2269–71.
2. Visser N. Hurricane Sandy's impact, by the numbers (INFOGRAPHIC). Huffington Post. 2013. Available at: http://www.huffingtonpost.com/2013/10/29/hurricane-sandy-impact-infographic_n_4171243.html. Accessed December 15, 2013.
3. Roper William L, Boulton Matthew L, Caine Virginia A, et al. Deaths associated with Hurricane Sandy — October–November 2012. Centers for Disease Control and Prevention. Atlanta (GA): Centers for Disease Control and Prevention; 2013. Available at: http://www.cdc.gov/mmwr/preview/mmwrhtml/mm6220a1.htm. Accessed December 15, 2013.
4. Abramson DM, Redlener I. Hurricane Sandy: lessons learned, again. Disaster Med Public Health Prep 2012;6(4):328–9.
5. Anthony Antonacci & Dennis Connors. "Executive committee." Presented on November 28, 2012. Microsoft PowerPoint File.

Disaster Ethics
Shifting Priorities in an Unstable and Dangerous Environment

Valerie Bridget Satkoske, MSW, PhD[a], David A. Kappel, MD[b],
Michael A. DeVita, MD, FRCP[c],*

KEYWORDS

- Disaster ethics • Emergency medicine • Critical care medicine • Informed consent
- Life-sustaining treatment • Disaster medicine

KEY POINTS

- Caring for patients injured or sickened by mass violence or injury, natural disaster, or pandemic infections may present clinicians with unique ethical challenges.
- Disaster care medicine may require clinicians to reconceptualize how to fairly and compassionately distribute medical goods and services.
- Even with proper disaster preparedness, clinicians may experience moral distress when faced with deciding which patients will or will not receive potentially life-saving resources.

INTRODUCTION

Both emergency and critical care medicine are fraught with ethically challenging decision making for clinicians, patients, and families. Time and resource constraints, decisionally-impaired patients, and emotionally overwhelmed family members can make obtaining informed consent, discussing the withholding or withdrawing of life-sustaining treatments, and respecting patient values and preferences difficult. When the illness or trauma is secondary to disaster, the ethical considerations increase and change based on the number of casualties, the type of disaster, and the anticipated life cycle of the crisis. There is not an ethical one-size-fits-all response to disaster situations. Disasters create unique medical preparedness and response needs. Importantly, they also require ethical thought and preparation concerning issues, such as just resource allocation, public health concerns, limits on individual autonomy, and danger to providers.[1] This article considers the ethical issues that arise when health providers are confronted with the challenges of caring for victims of disaster, especially when

[a] Wheeling Hospital, 64 Medical Center Drive, Room 1168D, Health Sciences North, Morgantown, WV 26506-9022, USA; [b] WVOEMS, West Virginia State Trauma System, 1 Medical Park, Wheeling, WV 26003, USA; [c] Harlem Hospital, 506 Lenox Avenue New, New York, NY 10037, USA
* Corresponding author.
E-mail address: michael.devita@nychhc.org

Crit Care Clin 35 (2019) 717–725
https://doi.org/10.1016/j.ccc.2019.06.006
0749-0704/19/© 2019 Elsevier Inc. All rights reserved.

available resources are overwhelmed. Benefits of preparation and protocolization of these considerations to health providers, patients, and the public are discussed; attention to ethical considerations as the care plan is created can reduce the number of deaths and caregiver and patient moral distress. This planning can reduce the inconsistency of in-the-moment decision making, which can undermine public trust and transparency.

PRINCIPLISM AND THEORIES OF JUSTICE

Caring for patients who have been injured or sickened by mass violence or injury, natural disaster, or pandemic infections may present clinicians with situations that they seldom have, if ever, previously encountered. Because situational considerations may shift, situational ethical analyses need to be reevaluated in times of public health emergencies and disaster. Health providers have an obligation to anticipate ethical issues that may arise in such situations, to develop ethically appropriate clinical pathways and protocols, and to infuse disaster preparation and management with a transparent accounting of how decisions will be made and the foundational ethical principles on which they are based.[2–6] Principlism is an approach to biomedical ethics that uses a framework of principles—autonomy, beneficence, nonmaleficence, and justice—to identify and consider ethical issues/conflicts.[7] In day-to-day bedside medical practice, ethical discussions generally revolve around issues of autonomy, beneficence, and nonmaleficence. Justice concerns are relegated far away from the bedside to discussions of universal health care and public health issues. In a disaster, the paradigm shifts dramatically. Health providers and systems often are overwhelmed; how to allocate resources is the issue, and triage of patients must occur.[3] Justice concerns may supersede the autonomous decision-making rights of the individual patient (and perhaps the provider).[8]

Justice decisions affect access to health care on global, national, state, community, institutional, and individual provider levels every day. Decision rules have been designed regarding who has access to health insurance, how solid organs are allocated for transplant, and even who will be seen next in the emergency department. These rules rest on the fair distribution of health care goods and services. The rules governing the bedside decisions are typically (and best) created far from the bedside even though they govern the resource distribution for each patient and they are implemented at the bedside. A full exploration of justice issues in the routine health care setting is beyond the scope of this article. Instead, the article focuses on how the scarcity of health care goods and resources in times of disaster force promoting justice considerations so that the focus if shifted from autonomy to justice as a more relevant and essential ethical decision-making guide.[7,9–11] It is not only a utilitarian argument (best for the most) but also a justice argument (fairly allocating resources) that must be considered.

In triage, the objective is to distribute health care goods and services in the most effective, efficient, and equitable way possible. Triage in a scarce resource setting depends on the principle of utility, which requires doing the most good for the greatest number. In day-to-day practice in a setting of relative abundance of resources, however, triage relies more on the principle of to each according to need. In other words, when resources are available, patients often are prioritized according to who is most medically in need of the resources. So if there is enough for everyone, then as many people as possible should be saved by treating the sickest first. Ethical calculus changes, however, in times of scarcity.[2,3,10,12,13] In many disaster scenarios, the volume of patients and the severity of their medical needs overwhelm available health resources (space, personnel, supplies, and time), requiring health professionals to shift from an autonomy focused, 1 patient–1 provider, shared decision-making model to a utilitarian model, which seeks to minimize the suffering and maximize the benefit of as many people as possible with the available resources. Decisions may need to be made in the absence of informed consent conversations to facilitate efficiently resolving issues. This circumvention of autonomy is justified by the need to give proper care rapidly, based on the principle of beneficence. This already happens daily in the emergency department, where life-saving care may be rendered (beneficence) before consent because the pause in care may inflict harm (nonmaleficence). In worst-case disaster scenarios, those most in need, who require the highest number of resources, may be least likely to receive treatment, because they would consume a disproportionate amount of the resources without a proportionate likelihood of benefit.[14] These decisions are difficult to make on the fly. Even more difficult is to make the same decision across the disaster setting and clinicians. This exemplifies the justice concern: treating people with similar conditions similarly. Thus, ethical weight is shifted; justice concerns may outweigh autonomous decision-making rights. Some individuals may get less in support of doing the most good for the greatest number.[5] Moreover, applying the decision rules equitably is essential.

DISASTERS AND ETHICAL CHALLENGES TO SYSTEMS AS USUAL (ORGANIZATIONAL ETHICS)

As disasters unfold, the ethical focus of most health care systems, maximum care of the individual patient, must convert to a predetermined crisis standard of care model.[15,16] The standard of care model of necessity has an impact on both internal and external health delivery systems and triage at all levels, including scene, emergency department, operating rooms, ancillary services, and critical care units. The day-to-day role of all health care providers shifts, as do their responsibilities in terms of their duties to communicate and engage in shared decision making with individual patients and/or their surrogates, use best available resources, support family and community, and respect their professional and personal moral and ethical values. Generally expected communication and responsibilities to families and community may be significantly altered from the usual process of explain, recommend, and obtain consent. Time and policy/protocol limit the ability and need to interact with patients and their loved ones. In these situations, an explanation may be all that is possible, and perhaps, required.

Duty to Plan

The obligation to care for the health and well-being of patients is reflected not only in the codes of medical ethics but also in the principles of beneficence and nonmaleficence. A parallel obligation is assumed by elected officials and local community leaders to protect the health and welfare of the citizenry. Inherent in such obligations is the duty to anticipate and prepare for potential threats to the health and safety of a community and create plans to address those threats.[3,17] Jennings and colleagues[4] claim, "because planners will not be able to deliberate in a serious or sustained way about justice in the thick of a disaster, they should be asking ahead of time what sorts of responses are ideally (or at least adequately) just and which processes for decision-making are ideally or adequately fair and legitimate." Additionally, truth-telling and transparency regarding the goals of disaster preparedness, the decision-making process, and the principles and values that support both are required to build and maintain trust and demonstrate respect for persons.[2–4,9] This is not to say that high-quality on-the-fly frameworks cannot be created amid unique disaster situations. Recent situations in the news that demonstrated the need to apply quickly new ethical frameworks include the Chilean miners trapped after a cave-in, health care after tsunamis that crushed the social infrastructure in Asia, earthquakes in Italy and South

America, and Ebola outbreaks. Disaster workers benefited from borrowing from the preexisting ethical framework that was developed for disaster scenarios. The care delivery framework is dictated by the particular circumstances of the disaster.

Planning considerations

- How are triaging decisions going to be made, how are they going to be ethically justified, and who is going to be responsible for making them—both planning and real-time decisions?[2]
- How will internal and external communications flow, creating a hierarchy of communication needs and planned response? How will information be delivered to patients, families, and the community (in both a consistent and transparent manner before and during an event—to build and maintain trust)
- Possible unexpected disruptions to the plan must be entertained because disasters often unfold in unexpected ways,[1] not in a predictable evolution but at best a punctuated equilibrium,[18] thereby necessitating alternative pathways and recalibration[19] of the communication algorithm at each stage.
- What measures will be taken to ensure the safety of health care workers, and will they be prioritized for access to vaccines and other health services? Will their families be given priority as a form of reciprocity?
- Can the treatment be withdrawn from one patient for the benefit of another patient who has a better chance of recovery?
- How will providers recognize their moral distress? Will anticipation of critical incident stress and planning for postincident care be incorporated in the disaster plans? If so, who will be responsible for recognition and intervention during and after the event?[20]

In addition to these suggested planning considerations, there are many resources available to assist in disaster and pandemic planning and preparedness, such as those that appear on the Web sites of both the Centers for Disease Control and Prevention and the US Department of Health and Human Services.

Triage: conventional, contingency, and crisis

Conventional triage plans for multiple casualty incidents have been addressed in several disaster models, most of which fall into 4 main, color-coded categories: (1) green—those whose care may be managed in a delayed fashion on an ambulatory basis, (2) yellow—patients requiring immediate care but without demanding significant resources, (3) red—those patients who without extensive intervention would be expected to die but are likely to survive with appropriate care, and (4) black—those who are unlikely to, but might, respond to significant expenditure of resources as well as those beyond salvage.[5,21] Distinguishing those who require significant resources and who are likely to survive from those who are similarly injured but less likely to survive can be difficult, and the ambiguity can be distressing to all involved. On occasion, the criterion may be simply the resources required rather than the probability of survival. For example, one of the authors (MAD) recalls an event, while working in a refugee camp on the Thai-Cambodian border, when a baby with pneumonia was dying, and the majority of doctors insisted the baby be intubated, even though there were no ventilators to support the baby after intubation. The hope was to sustain the infant long enough to allow the patient to respond to antibiotics. One physician argued against it, but the others all agreed to take turns bagging the patient manually. They did that through the night, and in the morning, after each had taken their turns, they finally recognized that even people with survivable disease do not survive when resources are scarce. Neither the provision of ventilation nor the avoidance of ventilation was unethical per se but not intervening caused moral distress nevertheless. Knowledge that in another setting a person could be saved can make a triage decision to not intervene difficult for a triage officer and other caregivers and potentially increased their moral distress.[13] Standardizing and making known the rules for triage as well as the ethical principles underlying the rules can help disaster workers and those impacted by the disaster manage their natural distress.

Because it is so difficult and important, this disaster triage must be, and is, clearly described and rehearsed. In multiple victim scenarios that necessitate contingency plans to match and allocate resources to patients as they present, the rehearsal allows all the participants to engage cognitively in the procedural as well as the emotional and ethical aspects of the system. In a crisis, as resources become inadequate to meet the demand, there emerges a need for a dynamic, progressive, recurrent triage of patients already in treatment algorithms. The dynamic situation may of necessity require that patients be moved to different categories as the availability of resources changes and the response of patients to treatment becomes evident.[2,3,14,22,23] For example, a patient triaged "in" may be moved "out" if the probability of recovery changes or the need for resources for others increases such that there is an altering of the "in" criteria. This may entail difficult ethical decisions as providers consider withdrawing resources from one patient to provide to someone else with a better chance of survival and invoke a reexamination of the definition of the duty to care to one that is more global and less individualistic.[2] It is important to continue to make the implementation of the triage criteria equitable across all patients in the disaster, or else fidelity (trust) and justice are breached, undermining the ethical framework for the decisions.

As triaging decisions become more difficult and ethically complex (eg, triaging children, withdrawal of treatment not consented to, and shuffling or reallocation or resources) moral distress may increase.[3] For example, in an environmental disaster in an advanced health care environment, so called bridge therapies that prolong life long enough for other definitive therapies to be used are called into question. This is especially true for those that are time and staff intensive to utilize—such as ventilators, vasopressor therapy, pacemakers, and extracorporeal life support—may not be initiated or withdrawn based on resource consumption as much as for likelihood of survival.[2,13] It is possible that a patient on a ventilator prior to the disaster might be ethically removed once the disaster comes to pass because of the new setting: a disaster requiring a new ethical decision-making framework. Once a treatment plan has been started and the physician has entered into a therapeutic relationship with a patient, duties of beneficence, such as fidelity, may make withholding or withdrawing of care, especially with the intention to use for the benefit of another, seem a particularly egregious violation of the physician-patient relationship. It may seem to violate both the obligation to do no harm and a duty to care. The disaster changes the calculations. Communicating transparently planned and previously agreed-on policies, fair application of protocols, and discussion of limited therapeutic trial periods may satisfy providers' sense of fidelity to the individual patient.[2] It also is important to convey to patients and families that limiting of treatment options does not mean that care, comfort, and compassion will not remain priorities. As such, palliative care professionals should be included in disaster planning and response.[24,25]

These decisions are best made based on disaster protocols that supersede standard informed consent and shared decision-making models. A predefined triaging algorithm is invoked. The responsibility for decisions is transferred to a triage officer/physician based on predetermined protocol.[2,25] This is in no way to suggest that communication with patients and families should not be a priority in any disaster plan. Rather, when decisions are being made in such manner, it is extremely important to keep patients, families, health care teams, and the community informed of what the triaging protocols look like, the justice frameworks on which they were developed, and how to address challenges to triaging decisions.[2] Transparency and education before, during, and after a disaster are imperative to build and maintain trust at both the bedside and community levels.[26]

Duty to Steward: People and Resources in Both an Immediate Sense and Through Time

Stewardship requires the responsible planning and management of resources. To fulfill duties of stewardship, what the goals for those particular resources are and who stands to benefit must be understood. This article suggests that goals and priorities change in times of disaster. Disaster medicine care requires the plans for stewarding medical resources to change in order to satisfy in, a new ethical paradigm, the principles of beneficence, nonmaleficence, and justice.[15] Stewardship is usually thought of in terms of distribution of medical resources, such as beds, staff, medications, and equipment, but in long-lasting disasters or pandemic situations it may become necessary to consider triaging in terms of preserving societal and community stability. Planning for societal persistence after extreme events prompts the question: to what degree should medical triaging decisions consider preservation of societal infrastructure, population, and quality of life for survivors and future generations.[12,27] In general, respect for persons and equal rights make it ethically difficult to distribute health care goods and services based on social worth criteria when social worth is based on "inherent worth by virtue of wealth, status, power or charisma."[7,12] Social worth may take on a new relevance if the societal infrastructure is critically destroyed. Recovery of society may require certain people with necessary skill sets to enable the collective good. In this setting, such considerations may become necessary.[7,12] For example, the Centers for Disease Control and Prevention suggests in times of pandemic a vaccine distribution prioritization scheme that ranks vaccine manufacturers at the top of the list with military personnel, health professionals, and those whose services would be required to maintain or restore societal infrastructure. Social worth can change based on the specifics of the setting. One of the authors (MAD) was in a disaster situation in a malaria endemic region. Given the choice between a physician and an entomologist, the team would have chosen having the latter, because more lives could be saved by preventing mosquito proliferation than could be saved with antimalarial care. Social worth in this setting was impacted by the disaster at hand. Although a full exploration of this macrolevel resource allocation is not provided in this article, it seems important to acknowledge the unique ethical issues that pandemic poses with its unknown duration, mortality rates, and contagion levels.

Duty to Care and Beneficence: Personal Risk to Providers (Families) and Issues of Reciprocity and Liability

Due care is taking appropriate care to avoid causing harm, as the circumstances demand of a reasonable and prudent person.[7] A duty to care creates a fiduciary responsibility on the part of the provider to act in the best interest of the patient. In times of disaster, it seems the duty to care becomes a duty to care for, or act in the best interest of, all affected patients—as a collective. This does not mean that the individual patient necessarily receives less care or that the provider abandons or is less concerned with the care of the individual.[24] Rather, in an attempt to respect and care for the whole of those in need, the provider's goal becomes to provide justly for all of the individuals within the whole. The focus remains to save as many individuals as possible, while taking into account probability of survival, the resources available, and the societal need for certain individuals to survive. Unfortunately, both the clinician and the patient may experience this as a violation of the usual 1-to-1 physician-patient contract as it is generally understood. Normal ethics support the claim that this is a violation of the ethical principles underlying health care. This creates moral distress on the part of the provider and feelings of abandonment on the part of the patient. Again, it must be recognized that the priorities of the ethical principles may be shifted in disasters, resulting in a shift in care delivery. Planning and honest communication about decision making and protocols hopefully will alleviate some of the distress and loss of trust.[24]

In addition to the inevitable moral distress clinicians may experience, health providers may find themselves at increased levels of physical, personal, and professional risk when practicing disaster medicine.[28] Clinicians who provide care for patients with a highly contagious and lethal virus not only put themselves at risk but also may put their families and friends at risk.[28,29] The health professionals who remained with their patients during Hurricane Katrina not only risked their own health and safety by remaining in a dangerous environment but also potentially harmed their families should they die. In addition, they also exposed themselves to legal liability for medical decisions made during that time. So, what are the limits of duties to care and how are clinicians who put themselves in harm's way protected and compensated?[8,30] There has been some legislative movement to construct a legal framework to recognize a need for additional liability protection for those providing care in a disaster that necessitates a blurring of credentialing, privileging, and normal resource availability combined with an alteration in the usual duty to care for the individual patient.[15] For example, most states have Good Samaritan laws protecting clinicians stopping at a local disaster from some legal liability, thus promoting the likelihood that qualified individuals might engage in volunteerism and stop to help. More work needs to be done and standardized across state and regional borders.[9] In addition, thoughtful consideration in the planning stages should be given to the possibility of a contractual arrangement with providers in extreme disasters/pandemics who are placing themselves (and sometimes their families) at greater risk than normally assumed under prevailing professional code(s) of ethics.[4,30]

SUMMARY

In extreme disasters/pandemics, when crises standards of care become the paradigm, the ethical considerations become shifted and perhaps even more complex. Careful consideration of the necessary shift from respecting the autonomy of the patient and provider as a primary ethical standard to a justice model seeking to provide equitable distribution or resources, resulting in the most good for the most people, must be a part of a comprehensive plan for these devastating events. Engagement of, and communication with, the public, who represent the potential future victims, must occur in advance. This is a foundation that enables a respect for persons and transparency to be carried through any future calamitous event. Duty to steward resources, duty to care for the greater good of society, must be framed in a plan agreed on through all levels of the population at large, governing bodies, and the health care system. The complexity and the potential for disruption of the social fabric of the human community require significant effort from all concerned under the duty to plan.

REFERENCES

1. Phillips SJ, Knebel A, editors. Providing mass medical care with scarce resources: a community planning guide. Rockville (MD): Agency for Healthcare Research and Quality; 2006. Prepared by Health Systems Research, Inc., under contract No. 290-04-0010. AHRQ Publication No. 07-0001.

2. Biddison LD, Berkowitz KA, Courtney B, et al. Ethical considerations care of the critically ill and injured during pandemics and disasters: CHEST consensus statement. Chest 2014;146(4_Suppl):e145S–55S.

3. Leider JP, DeBruin D, Reynolds N, et al. Ethical guidance for disaster response, specifically around crisis standards of care: a systematic review. Am J Public Health 2017;107:e1–9.

4. Jennings B, Arras JD, Barrett DH, et al. Emergency medicine public health preparedness and response. New York: Oxford University Press; 2013.

5. Aacharya RP, Gatmans C, Denier Y. Emergency department triage: an ethical analysis. BMC Emerg Med 2011;11:16. Available at: https://www.ncbi.nlm.nih.gov/pmc/articles/PMC3199257/pdf/1471-227X-11-16.pdf. Accessed January 16, 2019.

6. Connorton P. Ethical guidelines for the development of emergency plans. Washington, DC: American Health Care Association; 2014. Available at: https://www.michigan.gov/documents/mdch/Ethical_Guidelines_for_the_Development_of_Emergency_Plans_AHCA_428875_7.pdf. Accessed January 30, 2019.

7. Beauchamp TL, Childress JF. Principles of biomedical ethics. New York: Oxford University Press; 2013.

8. Simonds AK, Sokol DK. Lives on the line? Ethics and practicalities of duty of care in pandemics and disasters. Eur Respir J 2009;34:303–9.

9. Hodge JG, Hanfling D, Powell TP. Practical, ethical, and legal challenges underlying crisis standards of care. J Law Med Ethics 2013;41(suppl 1):50–5.

10. Mallia P. Towards an ethical theory in disaster situations. Med Health Care Philos 2015;18:3–11.

11. Ram-Tiktin E. Ethical considerations of triage following natural disasters: the IDF experience in Haiti as a case study. Bioethics 2015;31(6):467–75.

12. Hearns JD. Social utility and pandemic influenza triage. Med Law 2013;32:177–90.

13. Lin JY, Anderson-Shaw L. Rationing of resources: ethical issues in disasters and epidemic situations. Prehosp Disaster Med 2009;24(3):215–21.

14. Eyal N, Firth P, MGH Disaster Relief Ethics Group. Repeat triage in disaster relief: questions from Haiti. PLoS Curr 2012;4. e4fbbdec6279ec.

15. Hanfling D, Altevogt B, Viswanathan K, et al, Committee on guidance for establishing crisis standards of care for use in disaster situations, Institute of Medicine. Crisis standards of care: a systems framework for catastrophic disaster response. Washington, DC: National Academies Press; 2012.

16. Institute of Medicine. Guidance for establishing crisis standards of care for use in disaster situations: a letter report. Washington, DC: The National Academies Press; 2009. https://doi.org/10.17226/12749.

17. Erdtmann F. Summary of featured study from the National Academies of Science, Engineering and Medicine. Mil Med 2016;181(8):719.

18. Eldredge N, Gould SJ. Punctuated equilibria: an alternative to phyletic gradualism. In: Schopf TJM, editor. Models in paleobiology. San Francisco (CA): Freeman Cooper & Co; 1972. p. 82–115.

19. Larkin GK, Arnold J. Ethical considerations in emergency planning, preparedness, and response to acts of terrorism. Prehosp Disaster Med 2004;18(3):170–8.

20. Hamric AB. A case study of moral distress. J Hosp Palliat Care 2014;16(8):457–63.

21. Cone DC, Serra J, Burns K, et al. Pilot test of the salt mass casualty triage system. Prehosp Emerg Care 2009;13(4):536–40.

22. Frykberg ER. Triage: principles and practices. Scand J Surg 2005;94:272–8.

23. Rigal S, Pons F. Triage of mass casualties in war conditions: realities and lessons learned. Int Orthop 2013;37:1433–8.

24. Karadag CO, Hakan AK. Ethical dilemmas in disaster medicine. Iran Red Crescent Med J 2012;14(10):602–12.

25. New York State department of health and New York state task force on life and the law update ventilator allocation guidelines. Available at: https://www.health.ny.gov/press/releases/2015/2015-11-25_ventilator_allocation_guidelines.htm. Accessed January 16, 2019.

26. Garrett JE, Vawter DE, Prehn AW, et al. Listen! The value of public engagement in pandemic ethics. Am J Bioeth 2009;9(11):17–9.

27. Vaccination of Tier 1 at all pandemic severities. Centers for Disease Control and Prevention. Available at: https://www.cdc.gov/flu/pandemic-resources/national-strategy/planning-guidance/pandemic-severities-tier-1.html. Accessed January 16, 2019.

28. Singer PA, Solomon RB, Bernstein M, et al. Ethics and SARS: lessons from Toronto. BMJ 2003;327(7427):1342–4. Available at: https://www.bmj.com/content/327/7427/1342. Accessed January 16, 2019.

29. Grimaldi ME. Ethical decisions in times of disaster: choices healthcare workers must make. J Trauma Nurs 2007;14(3):163–4.

30. Eckenwiler LA. Ethical issues in emergency preparedness and response for health professionals. Med Soc 2004;6(5):235–40. Available at: https://journalofethics.ama-assn.org/article/ethical-issues-emergency-preparedness-and-response-health-professionals/2004-05. Accessed January 16, 2019.

UNITED STATES POSTAL SERVICE® Statement of Ownership, Management, and Circulation
(All Periodicals Publications Except Requester Publications)

1. Publication Title	2. Publication Number	3. Filing Date
CRITICAL CARE CLINICS	000 – 708	9/18/2019

4. Issue Frequency	5. Number of Issues Published Annually	6. Annual Subscription Price
JAN, APR, JUL, OCT	4	$243.00

7. Complete Mailing Address of Known Office of Publication (Not printer) (Street, city, county, state, and ZIP+4®)

ELSEVIER INC.
230 Park Avenue, Suite 800
New York, NY 10169

Contact Person
STEPHEN R. BUSHING

Telephone (Include area code)
215-239-3688

8. Complete Mailing Address of Headquarters or General Business Office of Publisher (Not printer)

ELSEVIER INC.
230 Park Avenue, Suite 800
New York, NY 10169

9. Full Names and Complete Mailing Addresses of Publisher, Editor, and Managing Editor (Do not leave blank)

Publisher (Name and complete mailing address)

TAYLOR BALL, ELSEVIER INC.
1600 JOHN F KENNEDY BLVD. SUITE 1800
PHILADELPHIA, PA 19103-2899

Editor (Name and complete mailing address)

Colleen Dietzler, ELSEVIER INC.
1600 JOHN F KENNEDY BLVD. SUITE 1800
PHILADELPHIA, PA 19103-2899

Managing Editor (Name and complete mailing address)

PATRICK MANLEY, ELSEVIER INC.
1600 JOHN F KENNEDY BLVD. SUITE 1800
PHILADELPHIA, PA 19103-2899

10. Owner (Do not leave blank. If the publication is owned by a corporation, give the name and address of the corporation immediately followed by the names and addresses of all stockholders owning or holding 1 percent or more of the total amount of stock. If not owned by a corporation, give the names and addresses of the individual owners. If owned by a partnership or other unincorporated firm, give its name and address as well as those of each individual owner. If the publication is published by a nonprofit organization, give its name and address.)

Full Name	Complete Mailing Address
WHOLLY OWNED SUBSIDIARY OF REED/ELSEVIER, US HOLDINGS	1600 JOHN F KENNEDY BLVD. SUITE 1800 PHILADELPHIA, PA 19103-2899

11. Known Bondholders, Mortgagees, and Other Security Holders Owning or Holding 1 Percent or More of Total Amount of Bonds, Mortgages, or Other Securities. If none, check box ▶ ☐ None

Full Name	Complete Mailing Address
N/A	

12. Tax Status (For completion by nonprofit organizations authorized to mail at nonprofit rates) (Check one)
The purpose, function, and nonprofit status of this organization and the exempt status for federal income tax purposes:
☒ Has Not Changed During Preceding 12 Months
☐ Has Changed During Preceding 12 Months (Publisher must submit explanation of change with this statement)

PS Form 3526, July 2014 [Page 1 of 4 (see instructions page 4)] PSN: 7530-01-000-9931 PRIVACY NOTICE: See our privacy policy on www.usps.com.

---

13. Publication Title		14. Issue Date for Circulation Data Below
CRITICAL CARE CLINICS		JULY 2019

15. Extent and Nature of Circulation			Average No. Copies Each Issue During Preceding 12 Months	No. Copies of Single Issue Published Nearest to Filing Date
a. Total Number of Copies (Net press run)			276	305
b. Paid Circulation (By Mail and Outside the Mail)	(1)	Mailed Outside-County Paid Subscriptions Stated on PS Form 3541 (Include paid distribution above nominal rate, advertiser's proof copies, and exchange copies)	155	180
	(2)	Mailed In-County Paid Subscriptions Stated on PS Form 3541 (Include paid distribution above nominal rate, advertiser's proof copies, and exchange copies)	0	0
	(3)	Paid Distribution Outside the Mails Including Sales Through Dealers and Carriers, Street Vendors, Counter Sales, and Other Paid Distribution Outside USPS®	63	84
	(4)	Paid Distribution by Other Classes of Mail Through the USPS (e.g., First-Class Mail®)	0	0
c. Total Paid Distribution (Sum of 15b (1), (2), (3), and (4))		▶	218	264
d. Free or Nominal Rate Distribution (By Mail and Outside the Mail)	(1)	Free or Nominal Rate Outside-County Copies included on PS Form 3541	43	25
	(2)	Free or Nominal Rate In-County Copies Included on PS Form 3541	0	0
	(3)	Free or Nominal Rate Copies Mailed at Other Classes Through the USPS (e.g., First-Class Mail)	0	0
	(4)	Free or Nominal Rate Distribution Outside the Mail (Carriers or other means)	43	25
e. Total Free or Nominal Rate Distribution (Sum of 15d (1), (2), (3) and (4))		▶		
f. Total Distribution (Sum of 15c and 15e)		▶	261	289
g. Copies not Distributed (See Instructions to Publishers #4 (page #3))		▶	15	16
h. Total (Sum of 15f and g)		▶	276	305
i. Percent Paid (15c divided by 15f times 100)		▶	83.52%	91.35%

* If you are claiming electronic copies, go to line 16 on page 3. If you are not claiming electronic copies, skip to line 17 on page 3.

16. Electronic Copy Circulation		Average No. Copies Each Issue During Preceding 12 Months	No. Copies of Single Issue Published Nearest to Filing Date
a. Paid Electronic Copies	▶		
b. Total Paid Print Copies (Line 15c) + Paid Electronic Copies (Line 16a)	▶		
c. Total Print Distribution (Line 15f) + Paid Electronic Copies (Line 16a)	▶		
d. Percent Paid (Both Print & Electronic Copies) (16b divided by 16c × 100)	▶		

☒ I certify that 50% of all my distributed copies (electronic and print) are paid above a nominal price.

17. Publication of Statement of Ownership

☒ If the publication is a general publication, publication of this statement is required. Will be printed in the OCTOBER 2019 issue of this publication.   ☐ Publication not required.

18. Signature and Title of Editor, Publisher, Business Manager, or Owner

STEPHEN R. BUSHING - INVENTORY DISTRIBUTION CONTROL MANAGER

Date 9/18/2019

I certify that all information furnished on this form is true and complete. I understand that anyone who furnishes false or misleading information on this form or who omits material or information requested on the form may be subject to criminal sanctions (including fines and imprisonment) and/or civil sanctions (including civil penalties).

PS Form 3526, July 2014 (Page 3 of 4) PRIVACY NOTICE: See our privacy policy on www.usps.com

Printed and bound by CPI Group (UK) Ltd, Croydon, CR0 4YY

03/10/2024

01040482-0019